TABLE OF CONTENTS

INTRODUCTION

An ounce of prevention is worth a pound of cure, and herein are the basics of staying well. "Preventive health" and "wellness" are two catchall terms we've been hearing for a while, and though they may have the ring of trendiness, the reality is that the best medicine really is prevention.

When you eat, you ingest substances that your body needs to build and repair tissue, to burn for fuel, and to use in the billions of chemical reactions that occur every second. Those substances become *you*—and that fact underscores the trite but true expression, "you are what you eat." With the possible exception of quitting smoking, good nutrition is the single most important ingredient in the recipe for preventing disease. Unlike family history—which is an unalterable determinant of your risk—the food you put into your body directly affects your health and is completely under your control. Simple diet and lifestyle changes can make the difference between wellness and illness (or life and death).

Experts tell us that half of all deaths are due to an unhealthy lifestyle, and two thirds of those deaths are related to personal diet. So there's a lot at stake when you cruise those glittering supermarket aisles full of tantalizing come-ons and temptations. And while eating right won't guarantee you a long, healthy life, it certainly improves your odds. With the knowledge gained from this book, you'll be able to make smarter choices about what to have on hand in the pantry and refrigerator.

We'll start with a review of basic nutrition and food preservation. Then we'll look at four powerhouses of nutrition and healing: garlic, vinegar, olive oil, and surprisingly—chocolate! We'll also look inside the pantry to discover the surprising health benefits of some common foods like apricots, cinnamon, honey, oats, and tea. Finally, we'll explore how healing herbs, like alfalfa, echinacea, milk thistle, nettles, red clover, valerian, and yellow dock, are used. With a few choice ounces of prevention, you and your family may be able to put off needing that pound of cure.

HEALING

FOOD
SECRETS

Publications International, Ltd.

ISBN: 978-1-68022-709-3

Manufactured in China.

8 7 6 5 4 3 2 1

A SOLID BASE: NUTRITION

When you eat, you ingest many different substances—amino acids, fats, carbohydrates, antioxidants, and many other intriguing compounds. Your body has special uses for most of them. These vital substances are called nutrients. Let's review the major ones.

WATER

Every part of your body relies on water. Without it, you wouldn't live long—four or five days at the most. Your blood, for example, is more than three-quarters water. Other body fluids, such as saliva and digestive juices, are primarily water, as is urine. You couldn't get rid of body wastes without it. Almost every chemical reaction in the body takes place in a water medium; water also lubricates and protects the joints, organs, nose, and mouth. Your body needs water so that when you get hot, you can sweat. The water you sweat off then evaporates on your skin, cooling you down.

So how much do you need to drink? Generally, you should drink six to eight cups of water a day. Although you can get by on less, drinking this much water is especially kind to your kidneys and colon because it helps flush toxins out of your body. When you drink a lot of water, the toxins can't hang around long enough to cause damage to your kidneys or cancerous growths in the colon. In fact, drinking plenty of water may be the simplest of all disease-prevention tips.

Why not just drink when you're thirsty? Because your body's thirst-o-meter isn't very reliable. You should drink about three cups more than your thirst tells you to. And as you get older, your body loses the ability to tell when it's thirsty, making it doubly important to drink water even when you don't crave a cool drink.

CARBOHYDRATE

Poor misunderstood carbohydrate. It suffers from an image problem. Seems it got a bad rap years ago as a calorie-laden horror, and it hasn't been able to shake that reputation. Nothing could be further from reality. The message may be getting through that fat is your biggest enemy, but unfortunately, "carbs" are still viewed with skepticism.

Carbohydrates, however, are your best friends. They are your body's preferred fuel. Both complex and simple carbohydrates are broken down in digestion to glucose molecules, which are absorbed into cells and burned as a power source. When we say "burned," we mean it quite literally. In fact, the amount of energy provided by food is measured by the amount of heat it produces when burned; these units of heat are calories. All carbohydrates provide approximately four calories per gram.

They may all have four calories per gram, but that doesn't mean that all carbohydrates are the same. There are actually two kinds of carbohydrate: *simple and complex.* Sugars are "simple" carbohydrates. They are closest to the completely broken down form your body uses as fuel. In fact, glucose itself is the simplest sugar. So the body converts sugar directly into usable energy. Pure sugar foods, such as hard candies and soft drinks, raise your blood sugar level and your energy level temporarily—sometimes called a "sugar high." However, the levels quickly drop below what they were before, in a rebound effect. This has been dubbed the "sugar blues."

Complex carbohydrates—found in bread, pasta, potatoes, rice, starchy vegetables, oatmeal, and dry beans—are the basis of a healthful diet. These complex carbohydrates are better than the simple sugars for many reasons. One reason is they are absorbed more slowly (good for blood sugar control), but their real advantage is they are found in foods that contain many other nutrients. Unlike sugars, which are either by themselves providing empty calories or worse, paired with tons of fat, complex carbohydrates are found in grain products and vegetables that provide many important vitamins and minerals.

A great deal of the credit for the preventive powers of complex carbohydrates goes to fiber—a certain type of complex carbohydrate found in whole grains, legumes, fruits, and vegetables. It seems strange that something your body rejects can be so important to your health, but that's just the case with fiber—the indigestible portion of carbohydrate. Your body can't break it down, so it passes right through the gut and on out as waste. Yet to do without it is to invite trouble.

Without fiber, the other substances in your intestines would just sit there, fermenting and stagnating. Any toxins from food or created by bacteria would have that much more time to be in contact with your intestinal walls. This exposure is thought to be at least one cause of colon cancer. Keeping things moving is a smart idea that helps prevent other diseases and conditions as well: constipation, diverticular disease, hemorrhoids, and varicose veins. And the sticky properties of fiber keep diabetes, heart disease, and obesity at bay.

There are two types of fiber: soluble and insoluble. Insoluble fiber is the type that probably comes to mind when you think of fiber. It's found in the wheat bran in most bran cereals. The fact that it doesn't dissolve in water is what makes it so beneficial. Instead, it soaks up water like a sponge. This softens the stool and increases its bulk, which puts pressure on the walls of the intestines and speeds the stool's movement through your body. Making a regular habit of eating foods high in insoluble fiber can all but eliminate the worry of constipation and hemorrhoids, and it almost certainly decreases your risk of developing colon and rectal cancers.

Soluble fiber may not be as well known, but it's just as valuable. As soluble fiber dissolves in water, it forms gummy gels. These gels bind with substances you'd just as soon get rid of such as bile acids. Remember the oat bran craze? Well, it wasn't so silly. Oat bran is rich in soluble fiber, and by binding with bile acids, it helps lower blood cholesterol levels. The higher your blood cholesterol level, the more it can help you. To make a difference, get in the habit of eating one or two low-fat oat-bran muffins or other foods high in soluble fiber every day.

By slowing the absorption of carbohydrates, soluble fiber also helps keep blood sugar on an even keel. Some people with diabetes are able to control blood sugar better by increasing the soluble fiber in their diet. For those battling the bulge, the extra bulk in the stomach and its delayed emptying help curb the appetite without adding calories.

PROTEIN

Protein is overrated. Although getting enough may be difficult in some areas of the world, it's rarely a problem in the United States and other developed countries. In fact, too much protein is our curse. Still, it is essential for growth, indeed for life itself. Protein is made up of amino acids your body uses to make body tissue and vital enzymes. There are nine essential amino acids you must get in your diet.

You need about 50 to 60 grams of protein per day, and that's not as much as it sounds. Consider this: A quarter pound of cooked meat provides about 20 grams of protein, and a glass of milk adds another 8 grams. Every slice of bread, or equivalent serving of starch, adds another 2 grams each. So you see how easy it is to get enough protein. Anyone who eats meat gets more than enough easily.

FAT

We all know fat is not our friend when we eat too much of it. If we could avoid it entirely it might make things easier, but fat is also essential to life. Linoleic and linolenic acids are essential fatty acids, and fat is needed for brain functioning and absorbing fat-soluble nutrients.

However, don't take those kind words as license to pig out. You need fat only in very small amounts, and as long as you include a small amount in your diet, you're probably getting plenty. If you're the average American, more than one third of your calories come from fat—much more than you need. That's partly because fat, at about nine calories per gram, provides more than twice the four calories per gram of either carbohydrate or protein. Research suggests that you'd be better off if less than 30 percent of your calories came from fat.

Cholesterol is not a fat, although it falls into the lipid category. It is a waxy substance, found in all animal fats. Like fat, it leads a schizophrenic existence: vilified, but essential to life. Cholesterol is needed to make vitamin D and the sex hormones and is a key ingredient in the protective covering around nerves. The danger comes from the cholesterol circulating in your bloodstream. There, it can be attracted to any vulnerable spots along the walls of the arteries, where blood clots form and calcium also gathers. This aggregate deposit, known as plaque, continues to accumulate, narrowing arteries until blood can no longer flow through. If this happens to an artery in your heart, it's a heart attack; if it happens to an artery in your brain, it's a stroke.

VITAMINS AND MINERALS

Vitamins and minerals are crucial to normal body functions and some of them may have a role in preventing our most deadly diseases, such as cancer and heart disease, among other not-so-deadly ones. Getting enough vitamins and minerals for normal metabolism used to be our primary concern, but we know now that certain vitamins and minerals may be beneficial in even greater quantities. Certain others can be deadly in greater quantities. The real trick is knowing which ones you need more of and which ones you need less of.

The following vitamins and minerals are ones you may not get in adequate amounts. There are dietary solutions for most, but some nutrients are difficult to get in the average diet and may require supplementation.

Vitamin A. Do you eat your five servings of fruits and vegetables per day? Surveys show that less than half of adult women meet the Recommended Dietary Allowance (RDA) for vitamin A, probably because they don't eat enough fruits and vegetables rich in beta-carotene—a precursor of vitamin A. Suboptimal intake could weaken your immune system.

Riboflavin. You don't drink milk either? Only one half of adult women meet the RDA for this vitamin. If you're included in this poor showing, it may be because you don't consume enough dairy products and enriched grains in your daily diet.

Vitamin B6. Again, women are at the greatest risk for not meeting their needs for this vitamin. The average intake is just over 50 percent of the RDA. Women on birth control pills seem to need more than average. Some men may fall short too, as may seniors of both sexes. If you fit into any of these groups, your all-important immune system may suffer for it. In studies, supplements of vitamin B6 have been shown to boost immune function in seniors. Vitamin B6 may do even more than keep your immune system running. Exciting new research has shown vitamin B6 protects the body from a buildup of the amino acid homocysteine in the blood. High homocysteine levels have been linked to an increased risk of heart disease.

Folate (folic acid). This is a red-flag nutrient if you're a woman taking birth control pills. Smokers and alcoholics may be low, too. All women trying to conceive should consider a supplement, since a low intake can cause birth defects in the first few weeks after conception. Even women not considering pregnancy might benefit from the protection folate seems to afford against a virus that can cause cervical cancer. Men aren't left out in the cold either. Like vitamin B6, folate is necessary to break down homocysteine, an amino acid associated with increased risk of heart disease. Research on 15,000 physicians has revealed that those with diets suboptimal in folate and vitamin B6 were three times more likely to suffer heart attacks than those whose diets were adequate in the two nutrients. The FDA recently has mandated that folate be added to flour and grain products along with the other B vitamins and iron already added.

Vitamin C. Such an easy-to-get nutrient shouldn't be in this category, but certain groups of people don't get enough, particularly those who skimp on vegetables and fruits. Smokers typically have low blood levels of vitamin C because their needs are twice those of nonsmokers.

Calcium. The trend toward drinking soft drinks instead of milk with meals is having an effect. Less than a quarter of adult women and less than half of young children meet the RDA for calcium. That sounds bad enough, but it's really worse. The RDA's 800-milligram recommendation for adults is seriously outdated and may not be enough in the long run. This prompted the National Institutes of Health to issue new recommendations—much higher than the RDA. If you want to keep up with the new recommended levels, it may mean supplements, because now all adults are urged to get 1,000 to 1,500 milligrams of calcium, about the same as teenagers. A recent study of postmenopausal women found that those who took a daily supplement of 1,000 milligrams of calcium reduced their bone loss by 43 percent.

Copper. No one is yet certain about the cost of ignoring this seldom-noticed mineral. Some studies have linked low copper levels to arthritis, high blood sugar, heart disease, and high cholesterol. If you're typical, you are not getting even close to the RDA for copper. And if you take megadoses of vitamin C (1,500 milligrams per day or more) you could be disrupting copper absorption and contributing to a copper insufficiency.

Chromium. Talk about a deficit. A government chromium researcher estimates 90 percent of Americans get less than the minimum recommendation of 50 micrograms per day. So the new focus on chromium is deserved but misdirected. Its value is not in weight loss but in blood sugar regulation. The rise in blood sugar that comes with age may not be inevitable, but a result of inadequate chromium in the diet as chromium is needed for insulin to work.

Iron. You can forget the information you learned from those old Geritol ads. They gave a generation the wrong impression that only older women needed more iron. Women in their child-bearing years who are menstruating and losing iron monthly are at risk for anemia. Less than one fifth of them meet the RDA for iron. Children are also susceptible, especially toddlers, preschoolers, and adolescents who are growing rapidly and whose diets are typically lacking in iron. Athletes and vegans (who eat no animal products) should also watch their iron intake.

Fatigue doesn't always signal anemia, and anemia isn't always due to an iron deficiency, so any suspicion should be checked out by your doctor, who can run the appropriate tests. To boost iron absorption, drink orange juice (or another good vitamin C source) when you eat meat. Avoid drinking coffee or tea at mealtimes, and never drink them at the same time you take a supplement that contains iron.

Magnesium. Three out of four people do not meet the RDA for magnesium. This has implications for many growth and repair jobs in the body, but it can also contribute to osteoporosis. Calcium gives bones their strength; magnesium makes them elastic—just as important for resisting breakage.

Zinc. If you're not a big meat eater you might be short on zinc, unless you happen to like oysters. Just six medium Eastern oysters give you five to six times the RDA. Otherwise, you probably get only about half what's recommended. You need zinc for literally hundreds of enzymes that trigger important reactions in the body. The lower levels of zinc that come with age may be one reason for an increase in infections in older people. Seniors given zinc supplements show improved immune response.

However, caution is in order here. Too much zinc can also impair the immune system as well as cause a copper deficiency and lower blood levels of the beneficial HDL cholesterol. If you take a multivitamin-mineral supplement, be sure it contains 15 to 30 milligrams of zinc. Avoid supplements with a megadose of zinc.

TO SUPPLEMENT OR NOT?

That truly is the question. Although nutritionists like to insist on "food first," that isn't necessarily the end of the story. With smart supplementation, you may be able to make a good diet better or at least provide a measure of insurance against a deficit, but don't expect supplements to do too much.

Supplements, by definition, are there to supplement a diet, not substitute for it. Pills can't provide you with the disease-fighting phytochemicals that are in foods. Moreover, they certainly can't make a high-fat, low-fiber diet a healthy one. Downing single nutrients in large amounts can be risky because of the interactions among nutrients. That's why a multivitamin-mineral supplement may be best for most people, with exceptions for certain key nutrients.

Who might benefit from supplements? You'll notice that unless they fall into one of the special categories listed, men as a group are noticeably absent from the roster that follows. However, men who do not eat a balanced diet and are worried about their nutritional status might also benefit from a multivitamin-mineral supplement. They're best off seeking out one of the new formulas especially formulated for men that contain no iron.

- Infants need a source of iron when they reach the age of six months. Breast milk provides very little, and by this time, their body stores are depleted. Fortified cereal or formula fills the bill. A fluoride supplement is also recommended to prevent dental decay.

- Children usually get what they need from their diet. If their eating habits tend toward long jags or if they are vegetarians, a multivitamin-mineral supplement can provide insurance.

- Pregnant women and women planning to conceive are good candidates for a multivitamin-mineral supplement. It's wise to be sure your nutrient levels are optimal before becoming pregnant. It's also important to meet your body's increased need for the vitamins B6, C, and D and the minerals calcium, copper, iron, and zinc.

- Breast-feeding women are also candidates. Although their increased nutrient requirements can largely be met by the extra food needed to meet their increased calorie needs, a supplement can help insure against depletion of the vitamins B6, C, and D, and the minerals calcium, magnesium, and zinc. Calcium needs may dictate a separate supplement.

- Vegans and children who are vegetarians may not get all the nutrients their bodies need. Most vegetarians are no more likely to need a supplement than anyone else, but the exceptions may be growing children and adult vegans (who also shun dairy and eggs in addition to meat, fish, and poultry). They may need other sources of vitamin B12, vitamin D, calcium, iron, and zinc.

- Seniors older than 50 years of age need more of some nutrients and less of others, so they shouldn't pop pills indiscriminately. They need more folate and vitamins B6, B12, and D, though the body may have its own mechanisms for filling the B12 and folate gaps. Some also think it's wise for seniors to up their intake of the antioxidant vitamins C and E and beta-carotene. Postmenopausal women almost certainly need a calcium supplement. Based on the latest National Institutes of Health recommendations, women in this group require 1,000 to 1,500 milligrams per day.

WHOLE FOODS AND PHYTOCHEMICALS

The word *phytochemicals* refers to protective compounds found in plants. They are neither vitamins nor minerals, for they are not essential to life, but they may hold the key to optimal health. Genistein in soy foods, polyphenols in tea, psoralens in celery, sulforaphane in broccoli, allylic sulfides in garlic, and ellagic acid in strawberries—these are just a few of the exciting discoveries.

Scientists are busy trying to identify these and other phytochemicals and to discover just what they do. The task is daunting. An orange alone contains some 150 phytochemicals that provide various benefits, such as cancer prevention, cholesterol-lowering properties, and heart disease protection. Some researchers have futuristic notions of isolating some of these chemicals and then concentrating them into a single super-duper protective cocktail. However, it's premature to be so optimistic.

To benefit from phytochemicals, you need only to start eating more fruits and vegetables. You've probably heard the call to eat five servings per day. That's just the beginning. The real goal, say experts, is to eat five to *nine* servings of fruits and vegetables a day. Until now, researchers have focused on the beta-carotene and fiber in fruits and vegetables as the reason for their protective effect, but maybe that's not all there is to it. Maybe they have something else in common. Enter phytochemicals.

Carotenoids, other than beta-carotene, have begun to receive more attention. A lot of the same foods rich in beta-carotene are rich in other carotenoids that appear to have anticancer effects as well. Lycopene is one of the most promising. An Italian study suggests that people who eat a lot of tomatoes may have less risk of cancers of the gastrointestinal tract. Tomatoes are rich in lycopene.

Of course, tomatoes are rich in vitamin C too. So what is "the good stuff"? Maybe fiber is part of the equation. Or maybe the protective effect works only when these substances are all combined in the exact way they are in tomatoes. Perhaps the idea of extracting out "the good stuff" is naive. Of course, if you just eat more fruits and vegetables, it won't matter what the answer is.

PUT IT ALL TOGETHER

Let's get down to business. Although there are many guidelines for healthy eating, the simplest and most comprehensive are what's known as the Dietary Guidelines for Americans, which are issued and periodically revised by the U.S. Department of Agriculture (USDA) and the U.S. Department of Health and Human Services. Think of these seven directions as the seven wonders of the nutrition world.

Eat a variety of foods. This may seem obvious, but it's probably the most important prevention tip you can remember. No one food is perfect. No one food has it all. You can be assured of obtaining the best possible array of nutrients, getting the most important of the yet unknown phytochemicals, and avoiding too much of a single natural toxin by eating the widest variety of whole foods you can.

Maintain a healthy weight. Notice this doesn't say "ideal" weight. That's because what's healthy for one person might not work for another. You probably know what weight feels best for you. If you're overweight, try to lose; obesity is a risk factor for many serious diseases.

Choose a diet low in fat, saturated fat, and cholesterol. Cutting down on fat and saturated fat can help you prevent a variety of illnesses, including heart disease, stroke, high blood pressure, diabetes, and probably certain cancers.

Cutting back on cholesterol is just a bonus. Only certain people are sensitive to its effects, and if you cut the other two, cholesterol usually takes care of itself.

HALT THE SALT; SPICE UP YOUR LIFE

Over time, your taste buds learn to prefer less salt, but you'll probably miss it at first. You can minimize the trauma to your taste buds by using these specialized blends you can mix yourself:

Poultry blend: lovage, marjoram, sage
Vegetable blend: basil, parsley, savory
Salad blend: basil, lovage, parsley, tarragon
Italian blend: basil, marjoram, oregano, rosemary, sage, savory, thyme
French blend: chervil, chives, parsley, tarragon
Barbecue blend: cumin, garlic, hot pepper, oregano

Choose a diet with plenty of vegetables, fruits, and grain products. Follow this advice and you'll find it easier to eat a low-fat diet, because complex carbohydrates replace the fat in your diet. If you take this advice to heart, you'll automatically take care of your fiber needs, too. Besides, you can't get those all-important disease-preventing phytochemicals if you don't eat fruits and vegetables.

Use sugars only in moderation. A diet filled with sugary junk foods is likely to be high in fat and short on nutrients. You may feel full eating this food, but your body receives minimal benefit. Furthermore, it's not good for your teeth and may rob you of chromium.

Use salt and sodium only in moderation. Again, its reputation exceeds reality. Most people don't have a problem with sodium, but because we don't know who among us is the one person in ten whose blood pressure is sensitive to it, it's recommended that everyone take it easy with the salt shaker. Avoiding processed foods as much as possible also helps.

If you drink alcoholic beverages, do so in moderation. This is a controversial one. No one wants to advocate a drinking habit, because there are those who cannot handle it, but it's true that many studies have shown one drink per day can be good for your heart. Red wine may be best of all because of the extra phytochemicals it contains.

A note of caution: alcohol carries calories with no nutrients, so moderation more than makes sense. In excess, it can damage the liver; in pregnant women, it can harm the fetus; and combining it with medications is dangerous.

FITTING IN MORE FIBER

Upping your intake of fiber can be easier than you think, and you already know the benefits can be great (reduced risk of heart disease and cancer to name only two). Boosting your fiber intake can go hand-in-hand with cutting back fat, as long as you do it right. Here are some tips for filling up with fiber.

*   Switch to the whole-grain version of the foods you normally eat: brown rice instead of white rice; potatoes with the skin instead of peeled; whole-wheat bread instead of white bread; whole-wheat or lupin pasta instead of semolina pasta; whole-wheat or buckwheat pancakes instead of regular; bran muffins instead of blueberry muffins; graham crackers instead of buttery crackers; and so on. Then try adding new grains: barley, millet, triticale, and quinoa for extra fiber.

- Start your day with bran—either a cereal or a low-fat muffin. You could be a third of the way to your daily goal if you choose your breakfast wisely.

- Make dried apricots, prunes, or other fruits a healthy addition to your cereal. Dried fruits are an excellent source of fiber.

- Opt for the whole fruit instead of juice whenever you can. Juicing removes most of the fiber, especially if the juice is pulp-free.

- Fruits with seeds are powerhouses of fiber; raspberries and blackberries are the richest in fiber, but strawberries, blueberries, figs, and elderberries are also chockful.

- Top your sandwiches with spinach instead of lettuce; add tomato or sweet peppers. Use your imagination, but get some fiber-filled veggies in your diet.

- Find new ways to add vegetables: Add lightly steamed vegetables to spaghetti sauce, layer vegetables in your casseroles, or add vegetable purees to soups, sauces, and casseroles.

- Top your salads with lentils, chickpeas, green peas, and florets of broccoli.

- Add wheat germ into any baked product you make: cookies, brownies, muffins, quick breads, and especially pancakes. You can replace one half to one cup of flour with wheat germ.

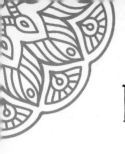

PRESERVING FOOD'S HEALING POWER

FRUITS AND VEGETABLES

You've heard it before and you'll hear it again—eat your fruits and vegetables! There is no doubt that a diet with plenty of fruits and vegetables offers a whole host of health benefits, including protection from heart disease, stroke, high blood pressure, some types of cancer, eye disease, and gastrointestinal troubles. It can even help beat back the effects of aging. Some fruits and vegetables are good sources of vitamin A, while others are rich in vitamin C, folate, and potassium. Almost all are naturally low in fat and calories, none have cholesterol, and many are great sources of fiber. Fruits and vegetables also add wonderful flavors, textures, and colors to your diet.

FIVE (OR MORE) A DAY

At a minimum, kids and adults should get five servings of fruits and vegetables every day—at least two of fruits and three of vegetables—but more can be better. People with higher calorie needs, such as teen boys and active men, should get about nine servings daily—four fruits and five vegetables. And for anyone wanting to cut calories and fat, extra servings of fruits and vegetables are excellent satisfying substitutes for higher-fat meats and sweets.

Here's what counts as a serving:

Fruits
- 1 medium piece of fruit
- ½ cup cut-up or cooked fruit
- ½ grapefruit
- ¼ small cantaloupe
- ¼ cup dried fruit
- ½ cup berries or grapes
- ¾ cup 100% fruit juice

Vegetables
- ½ cup chopped vegetables
- 1 cup raw leafy vegetables

- 6–8 carrot sticks (3" long)
- 1 medium potato
- ½ cup cooked or canned dried beans or peas
- ¾ cup vegetable juice

EAT A RAINBOW

If you haven't been eating much in the way of produce, choosing just about any kind of fruit or vegetable more often is a great way to start. But to get the biggest bang for your bite, think in color. Choosing assorted colors of fruits and vegetables is a great strategy for making sure you get the most nutritional value from your produce choices. In fact, an eating plan centered around colorful fruits and vegetables receives hearty endorsement from the National Cancer Institute, the American Cancer Society, and the Produce for Better Health Foundation.

In many cases, the deeper and darker the color of the fruit or vegetable, the greater the amount of nutrients it contains. For example, spinach offers eight times more vitamin C than does iceberg lettuce, and a ruby red grapefruit offers 25 times more vitamin A than a white grapefruit. Yet every fruit and vegetable has a unique complement of vitamins, minerals, fiber, and phyto-nutrients that provide benefits. So it's important to sample from the complete color spectrum as well as to eat a variety within each color group. Here are some ideas to expand your produce palette.

BLUE/PURPLE

These fruits and vegetables contain varying amounts of health-promoting phytonutrients, such as polyphenols and anthocyanins. The pigments that give these foods their rich color pack a powerful antioxidant punch. Blue and purple produce give you extra protection against some types of cancer and urinary tract infections, plus they may help boost brain health and vision.

Fruits
- Acai
- Blackberries
- Blueberries
- Currants, black
- Elderberries
- Figs, purple
- Grapes, purple
- Plums
- Prunes
- Raisins

Vegetables
- Asparagus, purple
- Belgian endive, purple
- Cabbage, purple
- Carrots, purple
- Eggplant
- Peppers, purple
- Potatoes, purple-fleshed

GREEN

Green fruits and vegetables contain varying amounts of potent phytochemicals, such as lutein and indoles, as well as other essential nutrients. These substances can help lower cancer risk, improve eye health, and keep bones and teeth strong.

Fruits
- Apples, green
- Avocados
- Grapes, green
- Honeydew
- Kiwifruit
- Limes
- Pears, green

Vegetables
- Artichokes
- Arugula
- Asparagus
- Beans, green
- Broccoflower
- Broccoli
- Broccoli rabe
- Brussels sprouts
- Cabbage, Chinese
- Cabbage, green
- Celery
- Chayote squash
- Cucumbers
- Endive
- Greens, leafy
- Leeks
- Lettuce
- Onions, green
- Okra

- Peas, green (or English)
- Peas, snow
- Peas, sugar snap
- Peppers, green
- Spinach
- Watercress
- Zucchini

WHITE/TAN/BROWN

White, tan, and brown fruits and vegetables contain varying amounts of phyto-nutrients, such as allicin, found in the onion family. These fruits and vegetables play a role in heart health by helping you maintain healthy cholesterol levels, and they may lower the risk of some types of cancer.

Fruits
- Bananas
- Dates
- Nectarines, white
- Peaches, white
- Pears, brown

Vegetables
- Cauliflower
- Corn, white
- Garlic
- Ginger
- Jerusalem artichoke
- Jicama
- Kohlrabi
- Mushrooms
- Onions
- Parsnips
- Potatoes, white-fleshed
- Shallots
- Turnips

YELLOW/ORANGE

Orange and yellow fruits and vegetables contain varying amounts of antioxi-dants, such as vitamin C, as well as other phytonutrients, including carotenoids and bioflavonoids. These substances may help promote heart and vision health and a healthy immune system; they may also help to ward off cancer.

Fruits
- Apples, yellow
- Apricots
- Cantaloupe
- Cape gooseberries
- Figs, yellow
- Grapefruit
- Kiwifruit, golden
- Lemons
- Mangoes
- Nectarines
- Oranges
- Papaya
- Peaches
- Pears, yellow
- Persimmons
- Pineapple
- Tangerines

Vegetables
- Beets, yellow
- Carrots
- Corn, sweet
- Peppers, yellow
- Potatoes, yellow
- Pumpkin
- Rutabagas
- Squash, butternut
- Squash, yellow summer
- Squash, yellow winter
- Sweet potatoes

RED

Phytonutrients in red produce that have health-promoting properties include lycopene, ellagic acid, and anthocyanins. Red fruits and vegetables may help maintain heart health, memory function, and urinary tract health and lower the risk of some types of cancer.

Fruits
- Apples, red
- Cherries
- Cranberries
- Grapefruit, pink/red

- Grapes, red
- Oranges, blood
- Pears, red
- Pomegranates
- Raspberries
- Strawberries
- Watermelon

Vegetables
- Beets
- Onions, red
- Peppers, red
- Potatoes, red
- Radicchio
- Radishes
- Rhubarb
- Tomatoes

FRESH AND BEYOND

There are lots of easy, nutritious, and affordable ways to enjoy fruits and vegetables all year long:

- Buy in season. Some types of fresh produce are great buys year-round, such as bananas, apples, broccoli, potatoes, carrots, cabbage, and spinach. Other items are more affordable—and better tasting—at certain times of the year. If your community offers a farmer's market, be sure to frequent it for extra-fresh produce.

- Go for convenience. Try prewashed and/or precut salad greens, baby carrots, and chopped fresh vegetables. The time savings can be huge, and the waste very little.

- Can it. Canned goods can be a low-cost, convenient way to enjoy your fruits and vegetables. Canned fruits and vegetables generally are comparable in vitamins and fiber to their fresh and frozen counterparts. Look for fruits packed in juice or water. Wash away extra sugar from canned fruits and extra salt from canned vegetables by rinsing them under cold water after opening.

- Hit the sales. Look for great deals offered by your local grocery store. Often, bargain prices on fruits and vegetables are used to draw in customers. Check the food ads before you shop. Since you're looking for variety, try the items that are on sale, even if some are new to you.

- Join the cold rush. Flash-freezing of fruits and vegetables keeps all the important nutrients locked in tight. Frozen produce is handy to keep in your freezer for whenever you may need it. Look for mixtures of vegetables to use in soups or stir-frys or to just steam or microwave and eat. Look for fruits frozen without added sugar.

IS IT RIPE YET?

When shopping for fresh fruits, you'll want to consider ripeness. As fruit ripens, the starch turns to sugar, which gives fruits their characteristic sweet taste. Some fruits continue to ripen after they're harvested, while others do not. Whether or not a fruit continues to ripen determines its storage and shelf life. For fruits that continue to ripen, it's a good idea to select them at varying stages of ripeness so they're not all ripe at the same time.

Fruits that require additional ripening should be stored at room temperature until they reach the desired ripeness. To hasten the ripening of some fruits, such as pears and peaches, put them in a loosely closed paper bag on the counter. They'll be ready to eat in a day or two. If fruits become overly ripe, instead of tossing them, try trimming any blemishes, then cooking and purée-ing the fruit to make sauces for dressings or desserts.

Fruits that do not ripen after harvesting should be stored in a cool area, such as the refrigerator, until you are ready to eat them.

Fruits that will continue to ripen
- Apricots
- Avocados
- Bananas
- Cantaloupe
- Kiwi
- Nectarines
- Peaches
- Pears
- Plums
- Tomatoes

Fruits to buy ripe and ready to eat
- Apples
- Cherries
- Grapefruit
- Grapes
- Lemons
- Limes
- Oranges

- Pineapple
- Strawberries
- Tangerines
- Watermelon

KEEPING YOUR PRODUCE NUTRITIOUS

Fruits and vegetables are naturally nutritious. It's how you store, clean, and prepare them that will determine how nutritious they are when you eat them. Fresh, properly stored produce will be the most nutritious. To keep produce fresh longer, store it unwashed and uncut. With the exception of a few items, such as onions, garlic, potatoes, and winter squash, fresh produce should be stored in the refrigerator. Most produce items are best stored loose in crisper drawers, which have a slightly higher humidity. If your refrigerator doesn't have a crisper drawer, use moisture-resistant wrap or bags to hold your produce.

Fruits and vegetables that have already been cut and/or washed should be covered tightly to prevent vitamin loss and stored on refrigerator shelves.

CLEANING

Wash your produce in clean water. This important step should be done for all fruits and vegetables, even for produce such as melons and oranges that have skin or rinds that you don't plan to eat. That's because surface dirt or bacteria can contaminate your produce when you cut or peel it.

Plan to wash your produce just before you're ready to eat or cook it to reduce spoilage caused by excess moisture. The one exception is lettuce—it remains crisp when you wash and refrigerate it for later use. It is not advisable to use detergent when washing fruits and vegetables. Produce is porous and can absorb the detergent, which leaves a soapy residue. Special produce rinses or sprays can help loosen surface dirt and waxes.

Clean thicker-skinned vegetables and fruits with a soft-bristled brush. Peel and discard outer leaves or rinds. If you plan to eat the nutrient-rich skin of hearty vegetables, such as potatoes and carrots, scrub the skin well with a soft-bristled brush. For cleaning fragile berries, such as strawberries, raspberries, blackberries, and blueberries, the best method is to spray them with the kitchen-sink sprayer. Use a colander so dirt and water can drain, and gently turn the fruit as you spray.

PREPARATION

There are plenty of ways to enjoy your fruits and vegetables. Eat them raw whenever possible to get maximum nutrition. For vegetables that require cooking, such as asparagus, green beans, or Brussels sprouts, cook as quickly as possible—just until tender crisp. This helps to minimize loss of nutrients and also helps vegetables retain their bright color and flavor. Cook vegetables (and fruits) in a covered pot with just a little water—to help create steam that speeds cooking. Or try cooking in the microwave. This fast method of cooking helps to retain nutrients, flavor, and crispness.

EASY WAYS TO GET YOUR HELPINGS

- Start your day with fruit—add fresh or dried fruit to cereal, yogurt, pancakes, or waffles, or just enjoy it alone.

- Mix chopped vegetables into scrambled eggs, or fold them into an omelet.

- First, freeze fresh fruits, such as grapes, blueberries, and chunks of bananas, peaches, or mango. Then, enjoy them as a refreshing snack, or mix them with yogurt and juice in a blender to make a smoothie.

- Snack on a trail mix of crunchy, whole-grain cereal, dried fruits, and chopped, toasted almonds.

- Bring a prepackaged fruit cup, box of raisins, or piece of fruit with you to work or school for an energy-boosting snack.

- For a shortcut fruit salad, open two or more cans of chopped or sliced fruit and add some fresh or frozen fruits for a tasty and refreshing snack or meal accompaniment.

- Stuff a pita pocket with veggie chunks and sprouts, and drizzle on a low-fat ranch dressing.

- Toss pasta or rice with leftover vegetables, lowfat vinaigrette, and a sprinkling of shredded cheese or toasted pine nuts or almonds.

- Sneak in some extra helpings of produce by adding finely chopped vegetables, such as carrots, eggplant, broccoli, or cauliflower, to marinara sauce, soups, stews, and chili.

- Roast your vegetables for a deep, rich flavor. Drizzle them with a little olive oil, and roast in an oven set to 425 degrees Fahrenheit or on the grill until tender. Try carrots, asparagus, butternut squash, eggplant, broccoli—or just about any vegetable that strikes your fancy!

BREAD, CEREALS, RICE, AND PASTA

This group of foods has one thing in common—they are all made from grains. Any food made from wheat, rice, oats, corn, or another cereal is a grain product. These foods should form the foundation of the diet for several reasons. First, grain-based foods are rich in complex carbohydrates, your body's best energy source. As the body's key fuel, carbohydrates provide your brain, heart, and nervous system with a constant supply of energy to keep you moving, breathing, and thinking.

Grain products also supply B vitamins and iron (especially if they're enriched or include the whole grain), as well as other beneficial phytonutrients (substances in plants with health-protective effects). In addition, many grain-based foods supply fiber.

THE "WHOLE" STORY

An important strategy for choosing the best grain foods is to seek out products made from *whole* grains. A whole grain is the entire edible part of any grain, whether it's wheat, oats, corn, rice, or a more exotic grain. The three layers of a grain kernel each supply important nutrients:

- The outer protective coating, or bran, is packed with fiber, B vitamins, protein, and trace minerals.

- The endosperm supplies mostly carbohydrate and protein and some B vitamins.

- The germ is rich in B vitamins, vitamin E, trace minerals, antioxidants, and phytonutrients.

When whole grains are milled (refined), the bran and the germ portions are removed, leaving only the endosperm. Unfortunately, more than half the fiber and almost three quarters of the vitamins and minerals are in the bran and germ. When you eat foods made from whole grains, you get all the nutritional benefits of the entire grain.

Enriched grain products add back some of the B vitamins—thiamin, folic acid, riboflavin, and niacin—and iron lost when the grain was milled. But lots of other nutrients and fiber don't get added back.

WHOLE GOODNESS

The individual nutrients in whole-grain foods—fiber, antioxidants, phytonutrients, and vitamins and minerals—each offer important health benefits of their own. When they work together in the "whole" food, however, they interact in powerful ways that help protect your health. For example, a diet rich in whole-grain foods is associated with lower risk for several chronic diseases and conditions including heart disease, cancer, diabetes, and gastrointestinal troubles. It can also play an important role in the treatment of many of these diseases.

A wide array of whole-grain foods is available in today's supermarkets. Examples of foods that can be found in whole-grain versions include breads, ready-to-eat and hot cereals, brown rice, pasta, crackers, tortillas, pancakes, waffles, and muffins. You just need to know what to look for.

YOUR DAILY GRAINS

You should get 6 to 11 servings of grains daily, depending on your specific calorie needs. Almost everyone should get at least six, and at least three of them should come from whole grains. A single serving of a grain food is equivalent to any one of these:

- 1 slice bread
- 1 ounce ready-to-eat cereal
- ½ bagel, English muffin, or bun
- ½ cup cooked cereal, rice, or pasta
- 1 four-inch-diameter pancake or waffle
- 1 seven-inch-diameter tortilla
- 5–6 whole-grain crackers
- 3 cups popcorn

Keep in mind that these are standard serving amounts—not necessarily the portions that you eat. Be sure to figure how many "servings" are in the portions you eat. You'll probably be surprised at how quickly grain servings add up.

GET YOUR WHOLE GRAIN'S WORTH

When you're choosing among grain products, follow these tips to get the most fiber- and nutrient-filled forms.

Breakfast cereals:
- Look for "whole grain" on the front of the package.
- The words "whole grain" or "whole" appear in front of wheat, oats, rice, corn, barley, or another grain as the first ingredient. Hint: Oats are always whole, even if they're rolled, instant, fine-cut, or coarse-cut.

Breads, tortillas, and crackers:
- Look for "whole wheat" or "whole grain" in the product's name.

- A whole-grain flour, such as whole-wheat flour, should be the first ingredient listed. Wheat flour, enriched flour, and degerminated cornmeal are not whole grain.

Pasta and rice:
- Only brown rice is whole grain.
- Look for pasta made from whole-wheat flour. Hint: Some pastas are made with a mix of whole-wheat and white flours; they may be a good stepping stone or compromise if you're having trouble adjusting to the texture of whole-wheat-only pastas.

YOUR DAILY BREAD AND MORE

Try some of these easy ways to make grains—especially whole grains—a regular part of your day.

- Get the first of your three daily servings of whole grains from a whole-grain breakfast cereal.

- Use whole-wheat pasta in hearty soups, hot casseroles, and chilled salads.

- Make the switch to brown rice, or try a combination of brown and white rice.

- When you make bread, muffins, biscuits, cookies, pancakes, or waffles, substitute whole-wheat flour for half of the white flour, or add some oats, wheat germ, or bran cereal.

- Take a whole grain to lunch—a sandwich on whole-grain bread is one way to go, or add some new appeal to your lunchtime meal with a whole-grain bagel, roll, tortilla, or pita.

- Snack on popcorn, lowfat granola made with whole oats, brown-rice cakes, or snack mixes made with whole-grain cereal.

- Sprinkle wheat germ, oat bran, or bran cereal on yogurt, salads, or cut-up fruit. Or use it to coat fish or chicken or to top a tuna casserole. When you prepare a meat loaf or any meat mixture, add some bran cereal or wheat germ instead of bread crumbs.

- Be adventurous and try whole grains you've never tasted, such as whole grain barley, bulgur, kasha, amaranth, quinoa, and couscous. Note: If you can't find whole-grain barley, choose scotch barley or pot barley, instead of pearled barley, which has lost a greater amount of fiber and nutrients in processing.

GRAIN STORAGE

All cereal should be stored in a dry location. Keep the inner bag folded down tightly to keep bugs out, or store the cereal in a container with a tightfitting lid. Once opened, it'll keep for a few months before it goes stale, unless you live in a humid environment. If so, your best bet is to not buy the large box unless you know you'll finish it in a month or so. Another option is to transfer the cereal to a resealable plastic bag and refrigerate it.

Keep oats in a dark, dry location in a well-sealed container to keep bugs out. Store the container in the refrigerator if you live in a humid locale. The oats will keep up to a year. Whole oat groats are more likely to become rancid, so be sure to refrigerate them.

Dried pasta is fine stored in your cupboards for months, especially if transferred to airtight containers. Putting your colored pastas in see-through glass jars makes a pretty display, but they'll lose B vitamins that way; better to keep them cool and dry, away from light, and sealed up tight. Rice and other grains are also best stored in a cool, dark location.

Brown rice is more perishable than white rice. It keeps only about six months—slightly longer if you refrigerate it.

Because of its fat content, wheat germ goes rancid easily. Always store opened wheat germ in the refrigerator in a tightly sealed container. If you buy it in a jar, you can simply store it in the refrigerator in its original container. Fresh wheat germ should smell something like toasted nuts, not musty. Unopened, a sealed jar of wheat germ will keep for about one year. Once opened, it can keep up to nine months in the refrigerator if the jar is resealed tightly.

Whole-wheat breads may not have preservatives added. To prevent your bread from going stale, leave out at room temperature only as much as you'll eat in the next day or two, and keep it tightly closed in a plastic bag. Put the rest in the freezer. It defrosts quickly at room temperature if you take out one or two slices as needed. Or you can defrost a few slices in a jiffy in the microwave. But don't refrigerate your bread—it actually goes stale faster.

MEAT, POULTRY, FISH, DRIED BEANS, NUTS, AND SEEDS

Foods in this group are diverse, but they have something important in common—protein. The amount and quality of the protein in these foods vary, but all are considered high-protein foods. The animal foods contain high-quality, or complete, proteins, which means they supply all the amino acids your body needs to build the proteins used to support body functions. The plant sources of protein supply lesser amounts, and the proteins are not complete; all of the amino acids are not found in a single source, although plant sources can be combined to provide the amino acids needed to form complete proteins. Besides protein, foods from this group supply varying amounts of other key nutrients, including iron, zinc, and B vitamins (thiamin, niacin, and vitamins B6 and B12). On the downside, some of the foods in this group contain higher amounts of fat and saturated fat. Some also include cholesterol.

HOW MUCH SHOULD YOU EAT?

Include two to three servings from this group—for a total of five to seven ounces—in your diet daily. Any one of the following counts as a single serving from this group:

* 2 to 3 ounces cooked lean meat, poultry, or fish
* 2 to 3 ounces lean, sliced deli meat (turkey, ham, beef, or bologna)
* 2 to 3 ounces canned tuna or salmon, packed in water

Other foods count as one ounce meat, or one-third of a serving from this group. These include:

* ½ cup cooked lentils, peas, or dried beans
* 1 egg
* ¼ cup egg substitute
* 2 tablespoons peanut butter
* ½ cup tofu
* 2 ½ -ounce soy burger

LEAN RED MEAT

Could it be that red meat—wonderful, juicy, stick-to-your-ribs red meat—might actually have healing properties, other than the obvious way it makes your taste buds and tummy come alive? Why yes, yes it could. But you must honor the word "lean" in front. And you need to cast meat as a bit player rather than the main character in your meals (sorry, but that means no more eating an entire 16-ounce steak in one sitting). Lean red meat, including beef, veal, and pork (sometimes erroneously referred to as "the other white meat"), can indeed be part of a healthful diet. And they can contribute nutrients that may help you maintain good health and prevent or even fight disease.

Beef, veal, and pork are packed with high-quality protein. They are also the most nutrient-dense sources of iron and zinc, minerals that many Americans have trouble getting. While it is possible to get enough iron or zinc without eating meat, it's not easy. Eating lean meat is also a dandy way to get vitamin B12, niacin, and vitamin B6. So, including some lean meat in your diet can be nutritionally uplifting.

The iron in red meat, especially beef, carries a double bonus. About half the iron in beef is heme iron, a highly usable form found only in animal products. And the absorption of the nonheme iron in meat is enhanced by the fact that it's in meat. Eating meat also enhances the absorption of nonheme iron from plant foods. (That's also a good reason to use smaller portions of meat mixed with plant foods in your meals.) The zinc in meat is absorbed better than the zinc in grains and legumes, as well. And despite the bad press red meat has sometimes received, recent research has shown that eating lean beef, veal, and pork is just as effective in lowering bad LDL cholesterol and raising good HDL cholesterol in your blood as eating lean poultry and fish is. Plus, close to half the fat in lean beef is monounsaturated, the kind that helps lower blood cholesterol and reduce the risk of heart disease when it replaces saturated fat in the diet. And the saturated fat that beef does contain is stearic acid, a form that doesn't appear to raise blood cholesterol the way other saturated fats do.

SELECTION AND STORAGE

The secrets to fitting red meat into a healthful eating plan are choosing lean cuts, trimming visible fat, preparing them without adding fat, and eating reasonable portions. When selecting red meat, here are some tips for finding the "skinniest" cuts.

Beef: Look for beef cuts with "loin" or "round" in the name, such as top round, round tip, top sirloin, bottom round, top loin, and tenderloin.

Veal: Lean cuts include cutlet, blade or arm steak, rib roast, and rib or loin chop.

Pork or lamb: Look for cuts with "loin" or "leg" in the name. Pork cuts include tenderloin, top loin roast, top loin chop, center loin chop, sirloin roast, and loin rib chop. Lamb cuts include leg, loin chop, arm chop, and foreshanks. You can also look for cuts labeled "lean" or "extra lean."

According to federal labeling regulations, cuts of meat labeled "lean" must contain ten grams of fat or less per three-ounce serving, and cuts labeled "extra lean" must contain five grams of fat or less per three-ounce serving. Don't be confused by ground beef labeled with a number followed by "percent lean." This refers to the weight of the lean meat versus the fat. For the leanest ground beef, simply look for ground beef that is at least 95 percent lean—it contains about five grams of total fat per three-ounce serving. Or look for ground round, which is the leanest, followed by ground sirloin, ground chuck, then regular ground beef.

When it comes to portions, forget the half-pound steak. To put a reasonable portion in perspective, three ounces of meat is about the size of your palm or a deck of playing cards. If you choose to eat all of your meat group servings at one meal, you can enjoy a steak that weighs about six to seven ounces or is about the size of two decks of cards. Or you can include a smaller portion of meat as a side dish and load up on vegetables and grains instead.

No matter the cut, choose meat that looks evenly red (grayish-pink for veal and pork) and not dried out. Refrigerate all meat as soon as you get it home. Place it on a plate so drippings won't contaminate other foods. If you don't plan to cook the meat within three to four days (one to two days for ground meat), freeze it.

PREPARATION AND SERVING TIPS

Defrost meat in the refrigerator, in the microwave, or sitting in cold water that you change every hour. Never let it sit out at room temperature, which invites bacteria to multiply.

Choose your cooking method to match your cut of meat. Some lean cuts, such as beef cuts from the round, do better with a method that includes a liquid, such as braising or stewing. Grilling, roasting, broiling, and panfrying work well for beef loin cuts. To minimize risk of foodborne illness, be sure ground meat is cooked until the internal temperature is 160 degrees Fahrenheit—or until the center is no longer pink and juices run clear. Roasts and steaks should be cooked until the internal temperature is at least 145 degrees Fahrenheit. Pork needs to cook to an internal temperature of at least 160 degrees Fahrenheit.

Trim all visible fat from meat before cooking. If you cannot buy ground meat as lean as you like, you can reduce the fat by placing cooked ground meat in a colander and pouring hot water over it. To tenderize tough lean cuts, try marinating, which also adds flavor, or do it the old-fashioned way and pound your meat with a mallet to break down the connective tissue.

POULTRY

Chicken and turkey are often considered healthy, lowfat alternatives to beef, but that's not always true. A piece of dark meat, such as a chicken thigh, with the skin on can carry a hefty fat load. You have to make the right poultry choices to really save on fat. Your best bet? Skinless white-meat chicken or turkey. It's lowest in fat and calories. Removing the skin before eating poultry saves fat and calories. But you quickly lose your lowfat advantage if you deep-fry it, smother it in fatty sauces or gravies, or cover it with cheese.

If you're trying to cut back on fat, skinless white-meat poultry offers a great lowfat protein option. You should be aware, however, that chicken and turkey contain about the same amount of cholesterol per serving as beef. Poultry is a generous source of some B vitamins that aren't as plentiful in beef, but it is only a fair source of iron.

Ground turkey is also available, but often it's higher in fat than you might think because it also contains ground turkey skin. For a truly lowfat ground turkey, look for "ground turkey breast."

SELECTION AND STORAGE

When choosing a whole chicken or turkey, look for one that is plump and firm with skin that looks moist and supple. The skin should have a creamy white or yellowish color (color varies depending on what the bird was fed), and it should have no odor. Poultry is a highly perishable food that presents a standing invitation to bacteria if it's not stored properly. If you buy a fresh, whole chicken or turkey, be sure to store it right away in the coldest part of your refrigerator and use it within two to three days. If you don't plan to use it within that time, wash it, dry it, cut it into parts, wrap it, and freeze it. It will keep for up to nine months. If you freeze it whole, it will keep for one year. Never let poultry thaw at room temperature. Thaw it in the refrigerator, and set it on a plate to catch drippings. It will take anywhere from one to two days to thaw a small 8- to 12-pound turkey, four to five days for a 20-pounder.

RECONSIDERING THE EGG

Eggs were once considered too high in cholesterol and fat to have a place on a heart-healthy menu. Many people still hold to the outdated advice to limit eggs to one or two a week. But unless you're following a very lowfat diet and your doctor insists on it, you can probably increase your weekly egg allowance.

Several years ago, scientists discovered that eggs contain less cholesterol than originally thought. This led to the old weekly egg allowance of one to two being upped to three or four eggs. More recently, experts decided that it would be safe to eat up to one whole egg per day.

It turns out that for most people dietary cholesterol has only a small effect in terms of raising blood cholesterol. Rather, it's saturated fat in the diet that has the greatest effect in causing blood cholesterol levels to rise. In studies where healthy participants ate up to one egg per day, there was no detectable effect on heart disease.

Although recommendations for strict limitations on eating eggs have been dropped, the American Heart Association still recommends keeping cholesterol intake to an average of 300 milligrams per day. One egg contains about 213 milligrams of cholesterol and 5 grams of fat, of which only 1.5 grams are saturated. So an egg a day can fit in a heart-healthy diet if your overall diet is otherwise low in cholesterol.

PREPARATION AND SERVING TIPS

When you handle raw poultry, be sure to wash your hands thoroughly afterward with soap and warm water before you touch any other food or utensil. Also be sure to wash well the cutting board and utensils used during preparation. Skip this important food-safety step and you're risking cross contamination—transferring bacteria like salmonella from raw poultry to other foods served at the meal. Cooking kills salmonella bacteria, but if the bug is transferred to a raw salad, for example, food poisoning can result.

If you marinate chicken or turkey, do it in the refrigerator, not on the kitchen counter at room temperature. And don't use the marinade as a sauce for the cooked bird unless you boil the marinade before serving.

Though fried chicken is an American favorite, especially the fast-food variety, it's also loaded with fat. Opt for lower-fat methods of preparation. Roasting is a good fat-saving cooking technique for whole chickens and turkeys. Skinless chicken or turkey breasts are perfect for marinating in lowfat sauces or, when cut up and mixed with vegetables, for stir-frying.

Chicken or turkey breasts also work well on the grill. If you want to add a sauce, wait until the poultry is almost done. Spread it on any sooner and it could scorch and burn before the breast is cooked all the way through. No matter how you prepare chicken or turkey, be sure it's cooked thoroughly to an internal temperature of 180 degrees Fahrenheit for whole birds and dark meat and to 170 degrees Fahrenheit for boneless roasts and breast meat—the meat should be white, not pink, and the juices should run clear.

Standard advice has long been to remove the skin of chicken or turkey before you cook it to save fat and calories. But it turns out that fat and calories are about the same whether the skin is removed before or after cooking. Since skinless poultry tends to dry out during cooking, keep the skin on while cooking to hold in moisture and flavor. Just remember to remove the skin and any fat left behind before eating.

FISH

Fish makes a fabulous addition to any healthy diet. Its generally low fat content (many types provide 20 percent or less of calories from fat) makes it a great protein option. And the fat it does contain appears to hold promise in terms of preventing and healing disease.

Eating fish instead of meat or poultry usually means less total fat, but it almost always means less saturated fat (as long as you're not ordering a deep-fried fillet and smothering it with tartar sauce). And that's important when it comes to the health of your heart and blood vessels. Ironically, though, fatty fish are better for you than lean fish, because they contain more omega-3 fatty acids. Two omega-3 fats, eicosapentaenoic acid (EPA) and docosahexaenoic acid (DHA), do a ton of good for your heart. EPA reduces the stickiness of blood platelets, preventing blood clots that can lead to heart attack and stroke. They also reduce triglyceride levels. DHA helps prevent irregular heartbeats by stabilizing electrical activity in the heart.

One study has linked omega-3s with less risk of sudden cardiac death. Another found that older people who eat just one serving of fatty fish a week are 44 percent less likely to die from a heart attack. And more recent research has confirmed the benefits of eating fish for both men and women. The Physician's Health Study of 22,000 men, for example, found that those with the highest blood levels of omega-3s had the least risk of sudden death. And the Nurses' Health Study of 85,000 women found two to four servings a week reduced heart disease risk by one-third. Even those who ate fish as little as one to three times a month showed benefits. As a result of much of this research, the American Heart Association now recommends two weekly servings of fish.

Omega-3s have also shown promise in easing symptoms of rheumatoid arthritis because of their anti-inflammatory properties. Again, adding fish to the menu just two to three times a week has been suggested as an adequate starting point.

You don't have to buy fresh to get the health benefits that omega-3 fatty acids offer. Canned fish, including tuna, sardines, and salmon, offer the same omega-3s as fresh varieties.

SELECTION AND STORAGE

Fish doesn't stay fresh long. If handled properly, fatty fish, such as bluefish, tuna, salmon, mackerel, or herring, lasts only about a week after leaving the water; lean fish, such as cod, haddock, or perch, lasts about ten days. To be sure the fish you buy is fresh, check for a "fishy" smell. If you detect one, don't buy it.

Whether you buy whole fish, fish fillets, or steaks, the fish should be firm, not soft, to the touch. The scales should be shiny and clean, not slimy. Check the eyes; they should be clear, not cloudy, and should be bulging, not sunken. Fish fillets and steaks should be moist; steer clear if they look dried or curled around the edges.

It's best to cook fresh fish the same day you buy it. (Fish generally spoils faster than beef or chicken, and whole fish generally keeps better than steaks or fillets.) But it will keep in the refrigerator overnight if you place it in a plastic bag over a bowl of ice. If you need to keep it longer, freeze it. The quality of the fish is better retained if the fish is frozen quickly, so it's best to freeze fish whole only if it weighs two pounds or less. Larger fish should be cut into pieces, steaks, or fillets. Lean fish will keep in the freezer for up to six months; fatty fish, only about three months.

PREPARATION AND SERVING TIPS

Preparing fish without adding lots of fat is simple. The key to keeping fish moist and flavorful lies in taking advantage of fish's natural fat and juices. The number one rule: Preserve moistness. In practical terms, that means avoiding direct heat, especially when preparing lean fish. You'll get the best results with lean fish, such as flounder, monkfish, pike, and red snapper, if you use moist-heat methods, including poaching, steaming, or baking with vegetables or a sauce that holds moisture in. Dry-heat methods, such as baking, broiling, and grilling, work well for fattier fish.

Fish cooks fast. That means that it can overcook quickly. You can tell fish is done when it looks opaque and the flesh just begins to flake with the touch of a fork. The general rule of thumb for cooking fish is to cook ten minutes per inch of thickness, measured at the fish's thickest point.

Marinades do wonders for fish. But as with poultry, keep safety in mind. Never marinate at room temperature; only in the refrigerator. And never use the marinade as a sauce for prepared fish unless you boil the marinade first.

LEGUMES (DRIED BEANS AND PEAS)

Legumes are a staple food all over the world. Dried beans and peas are one of the best sources of soluble fiber. Plus, they're low in fat and high in good quality protein—a great health-saving combination.

Beans can be gassy, of course, but there are ways around that. So don't let their "explosive" nature scare you away from some of the best nutrition around. The soluble fiber in beans helps lower levels of damaging LDL cholesterol in the blood, thus lowering heart-disease risk. And by slowing down carbohydrate absorption, soluble bean fiber fends off unwanted peaks and valleys in blood glucose levels—especially valuable to people with diabetes. Beans also provide substantial insoluble fiber, which can keep constipation and other digestive woes away.

Legumes are also rich in folic acid, copper, iron, and magnesium—four nutrients many of us could use more of in our diets. In addition, dried beans and peas are generally good sources of iron, which is especially helpful for people who don't eat meat.

SELECTION AND STORAGE

Most fresh nuts are available only in the fall and winter. Shelled nuts can be purchased anytime. Look for a freshness date on the package or container. If you can, check to be sure there aren't a lot of shriveled or discolored nuts. Be wary if you buy your nuts in bulk; they should smell fresh, not rancid. A caution: Aflatoxin, a known carcinogen produced by a mold that grows naturally on peanuts, can be a problem. Discard peanuts that are discolored, shriveled, or moldy or that taste bad. And stick to commercial brands of peanut butter. A survey found that bestselling brands contained only trace amounts of aflatoxin, but supermarket brands had five times that much, and fresh-ground peanut butters—like those sold in health-food stores—averaged more than ten times as much as the best-selling brands.

Because of their high fat content, you must protect nuts from rancidity. Nuts in their shells can be kept for a few months in a cool, dry location. But once they've been shelled or their containers opened, the best way to preserve them is to refrigerate or freeze them.

PREPARATION AND SERVING TIPS

When cooking with dried varieties of legumes, it's best to plan ahead. Before soaking or cooking, sort through the beans, discarding bad beans, pebbles, and debris. Then rinse the beans in cold water. It's best to soak your beans overnight, for six to eight hours; they'll cook faster and you'll get rid of gas-producing carbohydrates. But if you haven't planned far enough ahead, you can quick-soak for one hour. Quick-soak by putting the beans in water and boiling for one minute; then turn off the heat and let the beans stand in the same water for one hour. You may end up with a less firm bean, however.

After soaking, discard any beans that float to the top, then throw out the soaking water and add fresh water to cook in. Add enough water to cover the beans plus two inches. Bring to a boil, then simmer, covered, until tender—about one to three hours, depending on the bean variety. They're done when you can easily stick them with a fork. Remember, cooked beans double or triple in volume.

Beans are notoriously bland-tasting, but that's what makes them versatile. They can take on the spices of any flavorful dish. Add them to soups, stews, salads, casseroles, and dips.

NUTS

This category is just a little nutty. It encompasses some foods that aren't true nuts but have been given honorary status due to their similar nutritional qualities. These include the peanut (really a legume), the Brazil nut, and the cashew (both technically seeds). If you've relegated nuts to special occasions only, then it's time to reconsider. While they may be high in fat, nuts contain mostly mono- and polyunsaturated fats—fats with a heart-friendly reputation. In one study, people who ate nuts—almonds, cashews, pistachios, walnuts, or peanuts—five or more times a week were half as likely to have a heart attack or suffer from heart disease as people who rarely or never ate nuts. This protective effect may be attributable to the healthy fat profile of nuts, or it may be the result of the vitamin E and fiber found in nuts, both of which can help stave off heart disease; perhaps it's these several attributes combined and even other as yet unidentified ones that played a role. Other studies have demonstrated that adults with a high blood cholesterol level can lower both their total and LDL cholesterol levels by substituting nuts for other snack foods.

Besides being rich in protein, nuts offer a host of other nutrients, such as folate, phosphorus, magnesium, copper, zinc, and selenium. And another bonus—nuts are so dense with nutrients that they quell hunger pangs with fewer calories compared to other snack foods that often provide calories with minimal nutrition.

PREPARATION AND SERVING TIPS

To munch on as a snack, nuts are pretty much a self-serve affair. For nuts that are tough to crack, use a nutcracker or even pliers. A nutpick is useful for walnuts. Brazil nuts open easier if you chill them first. Almonds can be peeled by boiling them, then dunking them in cold water.

In cooking and baking, it's easy to get the nutritional benefits of nuts without overdosing on fat and calories, because a small amount of nuts adds a lot of flavor. Nuts sprinkled on your cereal can boost your morning fiber intake. Peanut butter makes a great snack on apple wedges or celery or simply spread on a piece of hearty whole-wheat toast. Walnuts go well tossed in Waldorf salad or with orange sections and spinach. Almonds dress up almost any vegetable when sprinkled on top.

Nuts give grains extra pizzazz and crunch. Pignoli, or pine nuts, add a dash of Mediterranean flavor when included in pasta dishes; they're the nuts you'll find in your pesto dishes. Nuts stirred into yogurt make it a more satisfying light meal. And spice-cake and quickbread mixes as well as pancake batters produce extra-special results when nuts are added in.

SEEDS

With their gold mine of healthy minerals and their niacin and folic-acid contents, tiny seeds are an excellent nutritional package. They are among the better plant sources of iron and zinc. In fact, one ounce of pumpkin seeds contains almost twice as much iron as three ounces of skinless chicken breast. And they provide more fiber per ounce than nuts. They are also good sources of protein.

Sesame seeds are a surprising source of the bone-building mineral calcium, great news for folks who have trouble tolerating dairy products. And seeds are a rich source of vitamin E. The only drawback: Some seeds are quite high in fat. Sunflower and sesame seeds provide about 80 percent of their calories as fat, although the fat is mostly of the heart-smart unsaturated variety.

SELECTION AND STORAGE

Seeds are often sold in bulk, either with their hulls (shells) in place or with their kernels separated out. Make sure the seeds you buy are fresh. Because of their high fat content, seeds are vulnerable to rancidity. If they're exposed to heat, light, or humidity, they're likely to become rancid much faster. A quick sniff of the seed bin should tell you if the contents are fresh or not. Seeds that still have their hulls intact should keep for several months if you store them in a cool, dry location. Seed kernels (seeds that have had their shells removed) will keep for a slightly shorter period of time.

Pumpkin and squash seeds are similar in appearance—both have a relatively thin hull that is white to yellowish in color. (Hulled pumpkin seeds are a popular ingredient in Mexican cooking.) Pumpkin-seed kernels are medium-dark green in color. Sunflower seeds are easily recognized with their hard black-andwhite-striped hull.

PREPARATION AND SERVING TIPS

You shouldn't go overboard with seeds because of their high fat content. But, in moderation, seeds can be mixed with cereals or trail mix or eaten by them-selves. A sprinkling of seed kernels over fruits, vegetables, pastas, or salads adds a touch of crunchy texture and flavor. Sesame seeds are especially attractive as toppers for breads, rolls, salads, and stir-fries.

MILK, YOGURT, AND CHEESE

Foods in this group supply approximately 75 percent of the calcium we consume. In addition, they provide protein, phosphorus, magnesium, and vitamins A, D, B12, and riboflavin. Although milk, yogurt, and cheese offer significant amounts of calcium and other key nutrients, most people eat only half the recommended daily servings from this group. That means many people—adults and children—may not be getting enough calcium and other nutrients essential to staying healthy. Certainly, foods from other groups contain calcium, but foods outside this group generally contain less, and the body may not absorb it as well.

CALCIUM FOR HEALTH

It is well known that calcium plays some pivotal roles in maintaining good health—from keeping bones healthy and strong and helping prevent high blood pressure to more recent findings that the calcium in dairy products may make it easier to lose weight. Calcium also helps your blood to clot and keeps your muscles and nerves working properly. If your body doesn't get enough calcium from food, it steals calcium from your bones to help keep a steady amount in your blood. Fortunately, it can be fairly easy to meet your daily calcium needs if you regularly enjoy milk, yogurt, and cheese.

THE SUNSHINE VITAMIN

Vitamin D is an essential nutrient for building and maintaining strong bones and teeth. It is a unique vitamin—your body can make its own vitamin D when sunlight makes contact with your skin. To get enough, it only takes a few minutes of sun exposure, three times a week, on your hands, arms, or face (without sunscreen). However, if you live in Northern climates or don't get outdoors much, especially in the winter, you shouldn't rely on sunshine. Also, as you age, your body may not be as efficient at making vitamin D, so food sources become even more important.

Your most reliable source of vitamin D is milk. Although milk is fortified with the vitamin, dairy products made from milk such as cheese, yogurt, and ice cream are generally not fortified with vitamin D. Only a few foods, including fatty fish and fish oils, naturally contain significant amounts of vitamin D. Other foods that contain smaller amounts of vitamin D include eggs, fortified breakfast cereals, and margarine.

SERVING UP DAIRY

To meet your calcium requirements, most people should have about three servings of dairy foods each day. Teens have the highest calcium requirements and should get about four daily servings.

Each of the following equals a serving of dairy:

- 1 cup milk
- 1 cup yogurt
- 1 ½ ounces natural cheese (cheddar, Swiss, Monterey Jack, etc.)
- 2 ounces processed cheese (American)
- ½ cup evaporated milk
- ⅓ cup dry milk
- ½ cup ricotta cheese
- 1 ½ cups frozen yogurt
- 2 cups cottage cheese
- 1 ½ cups ice cream
-

Note: For some of these, such as frozen yogurt, cottage cheese, and ice cream, a typical or reasonable portion is smaller than the amount that equals a single serving—for example, you're more likely to have only one cup of cottage cheese in a sitting—so count your actual portion for what it is, such as half a serving in the cottage cheese example. *Also note:* Other dairy-based foods, such as butter, cream cheese, and sour cream, are not considered dairy servings. These foods are made from the cream portion of milk and contain mostly fat and little, if any, calcium.

VERSATILE MILK

There are many varieties of milk—with different flavors and nutrition profiles. The easiest way to enjoy milk is ice-cold with a meal or snack. Most types of milk have about the same amount of calcium, protein, and most other nutrients per cup. The main differences are in calories and fat. Obviously, you're better off nutritionally if you choose skim, or at least 1 percent, milk to keep fat and excess calories to a minimum. However, if you have children under the age of two, give them whole milk. Young, rapidly growing children need the calories and fat that whole milk provides.

You might also want to give buttermilk a try. With its distinctively tart, sour taste, it's not for everyone, but many people prefer its flavor. Buttermilk is not as fattening as it sounds. Though originally a by-product of butter, today buttermilk is made by adding bacteria cultures to fat-free or lowfat milk. Read the carton to be sure you're getting the low- or nonfat variety.

Note: Buttermilk tends to be saltier than regular milk, however (a concern if you have or are at risk for high blood pressure), and it may not be fortified with vitamins A and D.

BEYOND STRAIGHT UP

There are other ways to include milk beyond drinking it plain:

- Many recipes call for milk, and in others, you can easily substitute milk for water. For example, use milk to make hot cereals; pancakes and waffles; soups; packaged potato, pasta, and rice mixes; baked goods; desserts; and drink mixes.

- Cereal and a cup of milk makes a good anytime snack—and it meets about a third of your daily requirement for calcium.

- Try blending milk with yogurt, fruit, and ice cubes for a refreshing fruit smoothie. Add a flavor twist by using chocolate-, banana-, vanilla-, or strawberry-flavored milk.

- Have some coffee with your milk. Try a café latte or cappuccino to get a healthy amount of milk with your coffee.

- If you're a soda drinker, consider choosing fat-free milk instead of regular soda once in a while to save about 90 calories and get milk's nine essential nutrients.

MILK STORAGE

All milk should have a "sell by" date stamped on the carton. This date is the last day the milk should be sold if it is to remain fresh for home storage. It does not mean that you need to use it by that date. Generally, if milk is stored in a closed container at refrigerator temperatures, it will remain fresh for up to a week after the "sell by" date.

Pasteurization—the process of rapidly heating raw milk, holding it for a short specified period of time, then rapidly cooling it—removes most of the bacteria from milk. However, some of the remaining harmless bacteria can grow and multiply, although very slowly, at refrigerator temperatures, eventually causing the milk to spoil. Store milk on a refrigerator shelf rather than in the door, which is not cold enough. To safeguard quality and freshness, store milk in the original container. Keep milk containers closed and away from strong-smelling foods. To avoid cross-contaminating milk, do not return unused milk from a serving pitcher to the original container. If milk has been left at room temperature for longer than two hours, throw it out.

Milk in plastic jugs is more susceptible to loss of riboflavin and vitamin A than milk in paperboard cartons. That's because light, even the fluorescent light in supermarkets, destroys these two light-sensitive nutrients. Today, you may find milk not only in the refrigerated section but also on the shelf with packaged goods. This is called UHT (ultra-high temperature) milk, referring to the processing technique. Though it must be refrigerated once you open it, unopened UHT milk will keep at room temperature for up to six months. UHT milk is just as nutritious as the milk you buy in the refrigerated section.

Drinking raw milk, or products that are made with raw milk such as some cheeses, can be risky. Raw milk has not been pasteurized and often carries bacteria that can make you sick. It's especially dangerous to give raw milk to children, the elderly, or people with impaired immune systems.

CHEESE, PLEASE

Cheese can be made from whole, lowfat, or skim milk or combinations of these. Regardless of the type of milk used to create it, cheese is a concentrated source of the nutrients naturally found in milk, including calcium. Indeed, many cheeses provide 200 to 300 milligrams of calcium per ounce. "Lowfat cheese" used to be an oxymoron. Not anymore! Today, there are dozens of reduced-fat, lowfat, and fat-free versions of American, cheddar, mozzarella, Swiss, and other cheeses, some you may find worth biting into. Fat in this new generation of cheeses has been cut anywhere from 25 to 100 percent. The average fat reduction is about 30 percent. Most of these contain added gums and stabilizers that help simulate the creamy texture and rich taste of full-fat cheeses.

The taste and texture of lower-fat cheeses varies considerably. Some people find them fine substitutes for the full-fat varieties, while other folks find they'd rather do without than settle for a lowfat substitute. Cheese connoisseurs will probably never be true fans of reduced-fat cheeses, but if you're trying to cut back on saturated fat and cholesterol, they do offer alternatives.

The one nutritional drawback of reduced-fat cheeses is that they are usually higher in sodium than full-fat natural cheeses. An ounce of regular Swiss cheese, for example, contains only about 74 milligrams of sodium. A reduced-fat Swiss may contain 300 to 400 milligrams or more per ounce.

Are reduced-fat cheeses the answer for a diet hopelessly high in fat? Hardly. Unless you're a big cheese eater, chances are other elements of your diet—such as fatty meats, whole milk, buttery muffins and croissants, chips, and ice cream—are more in need of a good fat-trimming. But substituting reduced-fat for full-fat cheese can't hurt. Another option for cheese lovers is to use strong-flavored cheeses, such as Parmesan, blue, or gorgonzola. With these, a little can go a long way in terms of adding flavor.

CHEESE SELECTION AND STORAGE

Many cheeses have considerably more fat per serving than a cup of milk. When shopping for lower-fat cheeses, here's what the label will tell you:

- Lowfat cheese: three grams or less of fat per one-ounce serving
- Reduced-fat cheese: 25 percent less fat than the same full-fat cheese
- Fat-free cheese: less than 0.5 grams of fat per one-ounce serving

For reduced-fat cheeses, opt for varieties that provide no more than five grams of fat per ounce. Regular cheeses provide eight to nine grams per ounce. Brands vary a lot in taste and texture. Shop around until you find one you like. You're better off choosing a reduced-fat cheese based on taste and then trying it in recipes. Remember, the less fat a cheese contains, the harder it is to use in cooking. Because of their high moisture content, lowerfat cheeses turn moldy more quickly than their full-fat counterparts. Keep them well wrapped in the refrigerator and use them as soon as possible.

COOKING WITH CHEESE

In general, the further you get from traditional cheese, in terms of fat content, the more careful you have to be about applying heat. It's the high fat content of regular cheese, generally about 70 percent of its calories, that gives full-fat cheese its smooth, creamy texture and allows it to melt easily. When you reduce the fat content, the cheese becomes less pliable and more difficult to melt. The lower the fat content, the tougher the melting problem becomes. Trying to make a cheese sauce with a reduced-fat cheese can truly be an exercise in futility because the product is prone to breaking down into a clumpy, stringy mess.

Nonfat cheeses are best served "as is" in unheated sandwiches or in salads. They generally have milder flavors than regular cheeses and sometimes have what cheese purists sometimes describe as slightly "off" flavors.

To lighten the calorie and fat load of recipes without dramatically altering the flavor or texture, try replacing one-half to two-thirds of a full-fat cheese with a reduced-fat variety. Grated cheese blends best. Or combine a small amount of full-fat, full-bodied cheese like extra sharp cheddar or Parmesan with a reduced-fat cheese. A little full-fat cheese can go a long way toward improving the flavor of the dish. Most reduced-fat cheeses melt smoothly when they are layered in a casserole; the layers serve as insulation and help prevent the cheese from separating or becoming stringy. The lower the amount of fat in a cheese, the longer it takes to melt and the more likely it is to produce a "skin" and scorch when baked. To counter this problem, top casseroles and baked pasta dishes with reduced-fat cheese only near the end of the baking time, and heat until just melted. Serve immediately.

Meltability on top of dishes like casseroles or pizzas varies among varieties of reduced-fat cheeses just as it does among traditional cheeses. You may, for example, find a fat-reduced mozzarella melts much more smoothly than a fat-reduced cheddar.

Meltability, texture, and taste may also vary among brands within a variety. Therefore, you'll probably need to do some shopping around and some experimenting to determine which varieties and which brands suit your needs and tastes in various situations; you'll probably prefer some kinds for snacking and other kinds for cooking or as toppings.

SAY YES TO YOGURT

Yogurt (along with some of its other fermented dairy cousins, like kefir) was a long-established staple in Eastern Europe and the Middle East before it reached our shores. And there was a time when yogurt eaters in this country were considered "health nuts." Our attitudes have changed considerably. Today, yogurt is commonly consumed by men, women, and children of all ages. Walk into any supermarket today, and you'll see the varieties and flavors of this nutritious food take up considerable space in the dairy section.

FRIENDLY BACTERIA

Yogurt may not be the miracle food some have claimed, but it certainly has a lot to offer in the health department. Besides being an excellent source of bone-building calcium, it is believed that the bacterial cultures, Lactobacillus bulgaricus (*L. bulgaricus*) and Streptococcus thermophilus (*S. thermophilus*), that are used to make yogurt carry their own health benefits. For example, research has suggested that eating yogurt regularly helps boost the body's immune system function, warding off colds and possibly even helping to fend off cancer. It is also thought the friendly bacteria found in many types of yogurt can help prevent and even remedy diarrhea.

For people who suffer from lactose intolerance, yogurt is often well tolerated because live yogurt cultures produce lactase, making the lactose sugar in the yogurt easier to digest. Be sure to check the label on the yogurt carton for the National Yogurt Association's Live and Active Cultures (LAC) seal. This seal identifies products that contain a significant amount of live and active cultures. But don't look to frozen yogurt as an option; most frozen yogurt contains little of the healthful bacteria.

YOGURT SELECTION AND STORAGE

There is a dizzying array of brands and flavors and varieties of yogurts in most supermarkets. But there are some basic traits to look for when deciding which to put in your grocery cart. Choose a yogurt that is either low fat or fat free. It should contain no more than three grams of fat per eight-ounce carton.

Some yogurts are also sugar free (these are often signaled by the term "light," but check the label carefully to be sure, since this term might also refer to fat content) and contain an alternative sweetener instead of added sugar. Consider choosing plain, vanilla, lemon, or any one of the yogurts without a jamlike fruit mixture added. The mixture adds mainly calories and little if anything in the way of vitamins, minerals, or fiber. Your best health bet is to add your own fresh fruit to plain fat-free yogurt.

Yogurt must always be refrigerated. Each carton should have a "sell by" date stamped on it. It should be eaten within the week following the "sell by" date to take full advantage of the live and active cultures in the yogurt. As yogurt is stored, the amount of live and active cultures begins to decline.

PREPARATION AND SERVING TIPS

Yogurt can be enjoyed as a lowfat dessert, snack, or meal accompaniment; just add sliced berries, nuts, wheat germ, bananas, peaches, fruit cocktail, mandarin-orange slices, pineapple chunks, lowfat granola, or bran cereal. Yogurt also works well as a lowfat substitute in a lot of recipes that call for high-fat ingredients such as sour cream or cream.

Yogurt is especially well-suited as a base for vegetable and/or chip dips and salad dressings.

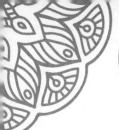

GARLIC: WORTHY OF THE HYPE

The wonders of garlic have been with us for millennia. Writings from ancient Egypt, Greece, India, and China all make mention of the humble garlic clove. It has long been used in many cultures to improve health or transform meals into delicious, aromatic delights. Its ability to enhance flavor is undeniable, while the extent of its healing benefits continues to be revealed.

In many historic cultures, garlic was used medicinally but not in cooking. That might surprise us today, but were our ancestors able to travel into the future to visit us, they would likely think us rather dense for our culture's general lack of appreciation for the bulb's healing qualities.

Traditionally, garlic bulbs were prepared in a variety of ways for medicinal purposes. The juice of the bulb might be extracted and taken internally for one purpose, while the bulb might be ground into a paste for external treatment of other health problems. In the minds of the superstitious, simply possessing garlic was enough to bring good luck and protect against evil or mysterious entities.

Garlic played its first starring role in modern medical treatment during World War I. The Russians used garlic on the front lines to treat battle wounds and fight infection, and medics used moss that was soaked in garlic as an antiseptic to pack wounds.

In the first part of the 20th century, garlic saw plenty of action off the battlefield, too. Even though penicillin was discovered in 1928, the demand for it among the general population often outstripped the supply, so many people continued with the treatments they had used with some success before, including garlic.

The pungent, ancient remedy has found its way to modern times. Herbalists have long touted garlic for a number of health problems, from preventing colds and treating intestinal problems to lowering blood cholesterol and reducing heart disease risk. Garlic remedies abound—and scientific research has begun to support the usefulness of some of them.

Garlic's popularity today is due in part to the efforts of scientists around the world. They have identified a number of sulfur-containing compounds in garlic that have important medicinal properties.

If you were to look at or sniff an intact garlic clove sitting on a cutting board, you'd never suspect the potent aroma and healing properties within. Whack it with a knife, however, and you open a portal!

Cutting, crushing, or chewing a garlic clove activates numerous sulfurous substances. When these substances come into contact with oxygen, they form compounds that have therapeutic properties. The most researched, and possibly the most medicinally powerful, of these potent compounds are allicin and ajoene.

A LITTLE HELP FOR YOUR HEART

The tiny garlic clove may play a big role in reducing the risk of heart disease, heart attacks, and stroke. How could such a simple thing have such powerful, far-reaching effects? To explore the answer and gain some appreciation for garlic's labors on our behalf, it's important to have a basic understanding of how the heart functions in sickness and in health.

Heart disease is the number one killer of Americans. The most common form of heart disease occurs when the arteries that deliver oxygen- and nutrient-rich blood to the heart become narrowed or clogged and lose their elasticity. Blood flow to the heart diminishes or may be cut off completely, starving the organ of oxygen. Without adequate oxygen, the heart can no longer work properly and heart cells begin to die.

Healthy arteries are similar to flexible tubes, wide open and able to contract and expand slightly as blood surges through with each heartbeat. When there is any injury to the inner lining of these vital tubes—such as damage caused by high blood cholesterol and triglyceride levels, high blood pressure, tobacco smoke, diabetes, and the aging process—the body tries to protect and heal the wounded area by producing a sticky substance to cover the damage.

This process is similar to the way we might use spackle to patch a small hole in drywall. But the sticky spackle the body produces to heal the wound causes fatty substances (including cholesterol), proteins, calcium, inflammatory cells, and other "debris" in the blood to stick to the vessel walls, forming plaque. As the plaque accumulates on the inner walls of the arteries, the arteries become less elastic, which leaves them vulnerable to even more injury. The gradual buildup of plaque also slowly narrows the inner diameter of the artery, and blood flow is hampered.

In addition, the plaque itself can crack, or bits of plaque can become dislodged. The body responds by sending platelets (particles in the blood that aid clotting) to form a clot around the plaque, further narrowing the artery. In some cases, the blood clot may completely block the flow of blood through the artery. Cells beyond the blockage that depend on a steady flow of oxygen from the blood can die. When this occurs in an artery that feeds the heart muscle (known as a coronary artery), it's called a heart attack. If this happens in a vessel that feeds the brain, the result is a stroke.

Some cholesterol is necessary for normal body processes—it is a vital part of cell membranes, transports nutrients into and waste products out of cells, and is part of the structure of many hormones, among other functions—but too much of the wrong kind leads to trouble.

When you eat cholesterol in food, as in meat, eggs, and cheese, your body breaks it down to digest it, then turns some of it back into cholesterol. Your body also makes cholesterol out of the solid fats (saturated fat and *trans* fat) in your diet. Heredity also plays a role in the amount of cholesterol your body produces. Genetics determine whether your body makes a little or a lot of cholesterol from the fats you eat.

GARLIC'S IMPACT ON BLOOD CHOLESTEROL LEVELS

You've probably seen advertisements for garlic supplements and debated whether you should eat more garlic to improve your heart's health. Perhaps you've wondered if it's worth the odor or if it's only good for keeping vampires at bay. Does garlic really promote heart health, and if so, how does it work?

Research on animals and humans in the 1980s and early 1990s seemed to indicate that garlic had much promise for lowering cholesterol. It appeared that garlic was able to lower total blood cholesterol in those who had high blood cholesterol (levels of 200 mg/dL or more). However, many of the studies included small numbers of patients and were short term, lasting just three months or less.

A number of more recent studies of garlic's healing properties have tempered the initial enthusiasm over its cholesterol-lowering effects. The National Center for Complementary and Alternative Medicine, a division of the National Institutes of Health (NIH), requested a thorough review of human studies that investigated garlic's ability to control cholesterol levels. The NIH released a paper in 2000 that concluded garlic did not alter HDL, but that it could significantly lower LDL cholesterol and triglycerides in the short term. Researchers determined that garlic had the greatest cholesterol-lowering effect in the first one to three months of garlic therapy. After six months, however, no further lipid reductions occurred.

Elevated cholesterol levels, however, contribute to heart disease over a long period of time. So based on this newer research, it would appear that although garlic may be a helpful addition to a cholesterol-lowering diet, it can't be relied on as the sole solution to high blood cholesterol levels.

Still, it's obvious that more research is needed. Indeed, the NIH statement in 2000 encouraged longer-term studies, as well as consideration of the type of garlic used. For example, there is some evidence that garlic must be cut or crushed to activate its health-promoting components. But the products tested in the various studies were not consistent. Some used raw garlic, while others used dried garlic or garlic oil; sometimes the raw garlic was cut, sometimes it was minced, and sometimes it was used whole. When dried garlic was used, it often was made into a powder and formed into tablets. It's also unknown whether garlic just stops being effective after several months or whether other factors in these studies influenced the findings.

DIFFERENT FORMS OF GARLIC YIELD DIFFERENT RESULTS

One of the difficulties in comparing studies of garlic's effectiveness in humans is that there are many different forms of garlic used in the studies. One may contain more of an active ingredient than another. For example:

Fresh cloves of garlic—chopped or chewed: These may impart the highest amount of allicin, but they have not been well studied yet.

Fresh cloves of garlic—swallowed whole: These showed no therapeutic value in a limited number of studies that have been done.

Dehydrated garlic powder—made into tablets or capsules: This form often provided some therapeutic value, but allicin content of these products varies within and among brands.

Enteric-coated garlic tablets: These are treated so they do not dissolve until they reach your intestines, rather than your stomach. Some studies show that enteric-coated tablets don't dissolve soon enough to release the allicin they contain. This type of tablet usually prevents garlic odor on the breath.

Nonenteric-coated garlic tablets: Tablets effective in studies were standardized to contain 1.3 percent allicin. These may be more effective than the enteric-coated tablets, but they do cause garlic breath.

Aged garlic extract: One of the active compounds in this form is ajoene. There have been conflicting results in studies of health benefits.

Garlic oil: Shows little therapeutic value in studies.

GARLIC'S ATTACK ON PLAQUE

Garlic contains several powerful antioxidants—compounds that prevent oxidation, a harmful process in the body. One of them is selenium, a mineral that is a component of glutathione peroxidase, a powerful antioxidant that the body makes to defend itself. Glutathione peroxidase works with vitamin E to form a superantioxidant defense system.

Other antioxidants in garlic include vitamin C, which helps reduce the damage that LDL cholesterol can cause, and quercetin, a phytochemical. (Phytochemicals are chemical substances found in plants that may have health benefits for people.) Garlic also has trace amounts of the mineral manganese, which is an important component of an antioxidant enzyme called superoxide dismutase.

ARTERIES

Arteries benefit greatly from the protection antioxidants provide. And garlic's ability to stop the oxidation of cholesterol may be one of the many ways it protects heart health. Garlic also appears to help prevent calcium from binding with other substances that lodge themselves in plaque. In a UCLA Medical Center study, 19 people were given either a placebo or an aged garlic extract that contained S-allylcysteine, one of garlic's sulfur-rich compounds, for one year. The placebo group had a significantly greater increase in their calcium score (22.2 percent) than the group that received the aged garlic extract (calcium score of 7.5 percent). The results of this small pilot study suggest that aged garlic extract may inhibit the rate of coronary artery calcification. If further larger-scale studies confirm these results, garlic may prove to be a useful preventative tool for patients at high risk of future cardiovascular problems.

EASING THE PRESSURE

Research suggests that garlic can help make small improvements in blood pressure by increasing the blood flow to the capillaries, which are the tiniest blood vessels. The chemicals in garlic achieve this by causing the capillary walls to open wider and reducing the ability of blood platelets to stick together and cause blockages. Reductions are small—10 mmHg (millimeters of mercury, the unit of measurement for blood pressure) or less. This means if your blood pressure is 130 over 90 mmHg, garlic might help lower it to 120 over 80 mmHg. That's a slight improvement, but, along with some simple lifestyle adjustments, such as getting more exercise, garlic might help move your blood pressure out of the danger zone.

THE BOTTOM LINE:
GARLIC AND HEART HEALTH

Garlic seems to deserve a spot on the battlefield in the fight against heart disease. Even if its lipid-lowering abilities are less extensive than once thought, it appears that garlic's antioxidant ability helps protect arteries from plaque formation and eventual blockage. Because garlic also appears to increase the nitric oxide in vessels and lower your blood pressure, it becomes even more valuable.

INFECTION FIGHTER

Garlic's potential to combat heart disease has received a lot of attention, but it should get just as much for its antimicrobial properties. Raw garlic has proven itself since ancient times as an effective killer of bacteria and viruses. Once again, we can thank allicin.

Laboratory studies confirm that raw garlic has antibacterial and antiviral properties. Not only does it knock out many common cold and flu viruses but its effectiveness also spans a broad range of both gram-positive and gram-negative bacteria (two major classifications of bacteria), fungus, intestinal parasites, and yeast. Cooking garlic, however, destroys the allicin, so you'll need to use raw garlic to prevent or fight infections.

One demonstration of garlic's antibacterial power can be found in a study conducted at the University of California, Irvine. Garlic juice was tested against a wide spectrum of potential pathogens, including several antibiotic-resistant strains of bacteria. It showed significant activity against the pathogens. Even more exciting was the fact that garlic juice still retained significant antimicrobial activity even in dilutions ranging up to 1:128 of the original juice.

OXIDATION

Oxidation is related to oxygen, a vital element to every aspect of our lives, so why is oxidation so harmful? Think about when rust accumulates on your car or garden tools and eventually destroys the metal. That rust is an example of oxidation. Similarly, when your body breaks down glucose for energy, free radicals are produced. These free radicals start oxidizing—and damaging—cellular tissue. It's as if your bloodstream and blood vessels are "rusting out."

Antioxidants destroy free radicals, including those that are products of environmental factors, such as ultraviolet rays, air pollutants, cigarette smoke, rancid oils, and pesticides. The body keeps a steady supply of antioxidants ready to neutralize free radicals. Unfortunately, sometimes the number of free radicals can overwhelm the body's antioxidant stock, especially if we're not getting enough of the antioxidant nutrients. When free radicals harm the cells that line your arteries, your body tries to mend the damage by producing a sticky spackle-like substance. However, as mentioned earlier, this substance attracts cholesterol and debris that build up within the arteries, causing progressive plaque formation. The more plaque in your arteries, the more your health is in danger.

Eating raw garlic may help combat the pathogens that get attack our bodies. Garlic has been used internally as a folk remedy for years, but now the plant is being put to the test scientifically for such uses. So far, its grades are quite good as researchers pit it against a variety of bacteria.

For eons, herbalists loaded soups and other foods with garlic and placed garlic compresses on people's chests to provide relief from colds and chest congestion. Now the Mayo Clinic has stated, "preliminary reports suggest that garlic may reduce the severity of upper respiratory tract infection." The findings have not yet passed the scrutiny of numerous, large, well-designed human studies, so current results are classified as "unclear."

Can a garlic clove help stop your sniffles? A study published in the July/August 2001 issue of *Advances in Therapy* examined the stinking rose's ability to fight the common cold. The study involved 146 volunteers divided into two groups. One group took a garlic supplement for 12 weeks during the winter months, while the other group received a placebo. The group that received garlic had significantly fewer colds—and the colds that they did get went away faster—than the placebo group.

Garlic also may help rid the intestinal tract of Giardia lamblia, a parasite that commonly lives in stream water and causes giardiasis, an infection of the small intestine. Hikers and campers run the risk of this infection whenever they drink untreated stream or lake water. Herbalists prescribe a solution of one or more crushed garlic cloves stirred into one-third of a cup of water taken three times a day to eradicate Giardia. If you're fighting giardiasis, be sure to consult your health-care provider, because it's a nasty infection, and ask if you can try garlic as part of your treatment.

Finally, in the January 2005 issue of *Antimicrobial Agents and Chemotherapy,* researchers reported the results of an investigation into whether fresh garlic extract would inhibit C. albicans, a cause of yeast infections. The extract was very effective in the first hour of exposure to C. albicans, but the effectiveness decreased during the 48-hour period it was measured. However, traditional antifungal medications also have the same declining effectiveness as time passes.

ANTI-INFLAMMATORY PROPERTIES

Inflammation is the body's reaction to an injury, irritation, or infection. The symptoms of inflammation include redness, swelling, and pain. Whenever the body suffers an injury, it sends many substances to the site to begin the healing process and to fight off foreign invaders, such as bacteria that can cause infections.

The body's ability to create inflammation is so powerful and effective that sometimes the surrounding tissues get damaged. This can occur at the site of a wound, inside blood vessels that have succumbed to an injury by oxidized LDL cholesterol, or in airways that are exposed to something that irritates them. Certain complexes in garlic appear to help minimize the body's inflammatory response. By decreasing inflammation, garlic may lend a hand by doing the following:

- Protecting the inside of your arteries
- Reducing the severity of asthma
- Protecting against inflammation in the joints, such as in rheumatoid arthritis and osteoarthritis
- Reducing inflammation in nasal passages and airways, such as that associated with colds

EXTERNAL TREATMENT

Garlic has many uses on the outside of the body, too. Applying a topical solution of raw garlic and water may stop wounds from getting infected. (Simply crush one clove of garlic and mix it with one-third of a cup of clean water. Use the solution within three hours because it will lose its potency over time.) A garlic solution used as a footbath several times a day is traditionally believed to improve athlete's foot.

A study conducted at Bastyr University, a natural health sciences school and research center near Seattle, showed that a garlic oil extract cured all warts it was applied to within two weeks. A water extract of garlic was much less effective, however. In the same study, the garlic oil extract also proved useful in dissolving corns.

Using garlic oil extract appears to work better than the old folk remedy of tying or taping a slice of garlic to a wart. If the slice of garlic is bigger than the wart or moves just a bit, it blisters the healthy surrounding skin (of course, you have the same risk when using wart-removing products that contain acid). Garlic's phytochemical compounds are strong enough to create chemical burns, so always apply externally with caution and do not use on young children. One way you can protect the surrounding healthy skin is to smear petroleum jelly on it before you apply the garlic.

CANCER CRUSADER

Some scientists think garlic may be able to help prevent one of the most dreaded maladies—cancer. The Mayo Clinic has reported that some studies using cancer cells in the laboratory, as well as some studies with animals and people, have suggested that eating garlic, especially unprocessed garlic, might reduce the risk of stomach and colon cancers.

The National Institutes of Health's National Cancer Institute drew similar conclusions after reviewing 37 studies involving garlic and sulfur-containing compounds. Twenty-eight of those studies indicated garlic possessed at least some anticancer activity, especially toward prostate and stomach cancer.

Because the studies in question were merely observational (they compared people who reported eating a lot of garlic to those who did not), more studies are needed. Still, the research the National Cancer Institute reviewed found that it may not take much garlic to reap these anticancer benefits.

Eating as few as two servings of garlic a week might be enough to help protect against colon cancer. Controlled clinical trials will help determine the true extent of garlic's cancer fighting powers.

What gives garlic this wonderful gift? Several factors, including antioxidants and those same sulfur-containing agents we've discussed before, including allicin. (Antioxidants help protect cells from damage; continual cell damage can eventually lead to cancer.) Allicin appears to protect colon cells from the toxic effects of cancer-causing agents. For instance, when meat is cooked with garlic, the herb reduces the production of cancer causing compounds that would otherwise form when meat is grilled at high temperatures.

Garlic's potential ability to decrease H. pylori bacteria in the stomach may help prevent gastritis (inflammation of the stomach lining) from eventually evolving into cancer. (H. pylori is most famous for its link to stomach ulcers, but it can also cause chronic gastritis.) Numerous studies around the world indicate that garlic's sulfur-containing compounds have the potential to help prevent stomach cancer.

GARLIC FOR WEIGHT CONTROL?

Studies performed on rats indicate that when fed allicin while on a sugar-rich diet, the rodents' blood pressure, insulin levels, and triglyceride levels all decrease. A study that appeared in the December 2003 issue of the *American Journal of Hypertension* showed other surprising results. The weight of the rats that were fed allicin either remained stable or decreased slightly. The weight of the rats in the control group increased. The researchers stated that, "allicin may be of practical value for weight control."

Certainly, additional research needs to be done into this possible action of allicin, but it again demonstrates how wide-ranging garlic's benefits could be.

GARLIC'S SAFETY

Garlic is safe for most adults. Other than that special aroma garlic lends to your breath and perspiration, the herb has few side effects. However, you should know about a few cautions:

- If you are allergic to plants in the Liliaceae (lily) family, including onions, leeks, chives, and such flowers as hyacinth and tulip, avoid garlic. People who are allergic to garlic may have reactions whether it's taken by mouth, inhaled, or applied to the skin.

- People anticipating surgery or dental procedures, pregnant women, and those with bleeding disorders should avoid taking large amounts of garlic on a regular basis due to its ability to "thin" the blood, which could cause excessive bleeding. Taking blood thinners such as warfarin (brand name Coumadin) or aspirin and other nonsteroidal anti-inflammatory drugs (such as ibuprofen or naproxen) along with garlic is not recommended unless you first discuss it with your health-care provider so dosing adjustments can be made. To be safe, if you have any questions about your use of garlic, talk with your health-care provider.

- Garlic interferes with medications other than anticoagulants. Garlic may interact with and affect the action of birth control pills, cyclosporine (often prescribed for rheumatoid arthritis), and some other medications. It also interferes with certain HIV/AIDS antiviral medications, reducing their effectiveness. Talk with your health-care provider and/or pharmacist if you take prescription medications and regularly eat large amounts of garlic or take any type of garlic supplement.

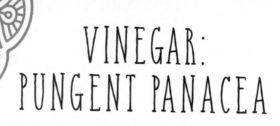

VINEGAR: PUNGENT PANACEA

Vinegar has been valued for its healing properties for about as long as garlic has, and like garlic, vinegar has found its way from the apothecary's shelf to the cook's pot. There seems hardly an ailment that vinegar has not been touted to cure at some point in history. And while science has yet to prove the effectiveness of many of these folk cures, scores of people still praise and value vinegar as a healthful and healing food.

Today, it can continue to play that dual role, taking the place of less healthful dietary ingredients and helping to regulate blood sugar levels while entertaining our taste buds with its tart flavor.

Fans view vinegar as an overall health-boosting tonic and recommend mixing a teaspoon or tablespoon of cider vinegar with a glass of water and drinking it each morning or before meals. (Apple cider vinegar is the traditional vinegar of choice for home or folk remedies, although some recent claims have been made for the benefits of wine vinegars, especially red wine vinegar. Unless otherwise specified, though, the vinegar we'll be referring to in the rest of this chapter is apple cider vinegar.)

Those who have faith in apple cider vinegar as a wide-ranging cure say its healing properties come from an abundance of nutrients that remain after apples are fermented to make apple cider vinegar. They contend that vinegar is rich in minerals and vitamins, including calcium, potassium, and beta-carotene; complex carbohydrates and fiber, including the soluble fiber pectin; amino acids (the building blocks of protein); beneficial enzymes; and acetic acid (which gives vinegar its taste). These substances do play many important roles in health and healing, and some are even considered essential nutrients for human health. The problem is that standard nutritional analysis of vinegar, including apple cider vinegar, has not shown it to be a good source of most of these substances.

HOW VINEGAR CAN HELP

So if vinegar doesn't actually contain all the substances that are supposed to account for its medicinal benefits, does that mean it has no healing powers? Hardly. We can't totally rule out many of the dramatic claims made for it. Although we know vinegar doesn't contain loads of nutrients traditionally associated with good health, it may well contain yet-to-be-identified phytochemicals that would account for some of the healing benefits that vinegar fans swear by. Scientists continue to discover such beneficial substances in all kinds of foods.

But beyond that possibility, there appear to be more tangible and realistic—albeit less sensational—ways that vinegar can help the body keep itself healthy. Rather than being the dramatic blockbuster cure that we are endlessly (and probably fruitlessly) searching for, vinegar seems quite capable of playing myriad supporting roles—as part of an overall lifestyle approach—that can indeed help us fight serious health conditions, such as osteoporosis, diabetes, and heart disease.

INCREASING CALCIUM ABSORPTION

If there is one thing vinegar fans, marketers, alternative therapists, and scientists alike can agree on, it's that vinegar is high in acetic acid. And acetic acid, like other acids, can increase the body's absorption of important minerals from the foods we eat. Therefore, including apple cider vinegar in meals or possibly even drinking a mild tonic of vinegar and water (up to a tablespoon in a glass of water) just before or with meals might improve your body's ability to absorb the essential minerals locked in foods.

Vinegar may be especially useful to women, who generally have a hard time getting all the calcium their bodies need to keep bones strong and prevent the debilitating, bone-thinning disease osteoporosis. Although dietary calcium is most abundant in dairy products such as milk, many women (and men) suffer from a condition called lactose intolerance that makes it difficult or impossible for them to digest the sugar in milk. As a result, they may suffer uncomfortable gastrointestinal symptoms, such as cramping and diarrhea, when they consume dairy products. These women must often look elsewhere to fulfill their dietary calcium needs.

Dark, leafy greens are good sources of calcium, but some of these greens also contain compounds that inhibit calcium absorption. Fortunately for dairy-deprived women (and even those who do drink milk), a few splashes of vinegar or a tangy vinaigrette on their greens may very well allow them to absorb more valuable calcium. Don't you wish all medications were so tasty?

CONTROLLING BLOOD SUGAR LEVELS

Vinegar has recently won attention for its potential to help people with type 2 diabetes get a better handle on their disease. Improved control could help them delay or prevent such complications as blindness, impotence, and a loss of feeling in the extremities that may necessitate amputation. Also, because people with diabetes are at increased risk for other serious health problems, such as heart disease, improved control of their diabetes could potentially help to ward off these associated conditions, as well.

With type 2 diabetes, the body's cells become resistant to the action of the hormone insulin. The body normally releases insulin into the bloodstream in response to a meal. Insulin's job is to help the body's cells take in the glucose, or sugar, from the carbohydrates in food, so they can use it for energy. But when the body's cells become insulin resistant, the sugar from food begins to build up in the blood, even while the cells themselves are starving for it. (High levels of insulin tend to build up in the blood, too, because the body releases more and more insulin to try to transport the large amounts of sugar out of the bloodstream and into the cells.)

Over time, high levels of blood sugar can damage nerves throughout the body and otherwise cause irreversible harm. So one major goal of diabetes treatment is to normalize blood sugar levels and keep them in a healthier range as much as possible. And that's where vinegar appears to help. It seems that vinegar may be able to inactivate some of the digestive enzymes that break the carbohydrates from food into sugar, thus slowing the absorption of sugar from a meal into the bloodstream. Slowing sugar absorption gives the insulin-resistant body more time to pull sugar out of the blood and thus helps prevent the blood sugar level from rising so high. Blunting the sudden jump in blood sugar that would usually occur after a meal also lessens the amount of insulin the body needs to release at one time to remove the sugar from the blood.

A study cited in 2004 in the American Diabetes Association's publication *Diabetes Care* indicates that vinegar holds real promise for helping people with diabetes. In the study, 21 people with either type 2 diabetes or insulin resistance (a prediabetes condition) and eight control subjects were each given a solution containing five teaspoons of vinegar, five teaspoons of water, and one teaspoon of saccharin two minutes before ingesting a high carbohydrate meal. The blood sugar and insulin levels of the participants were measured before the meal and 30 minutes and 60 minutes after the meal. Vinegar increased overall insulin sensitivity 34 percent in the study participants who were insulin-resistant and 19 percent in those with type 2 diabetes. That means their bodies actually became more receptive to insulin, allowing the hormone to do its job of getting sugar out of the blood and into the cells. Both blood sugar and blood insulin levels were lower than normal in the insulin-resistant participants, which is more good news.

Surprisingly, the control group (who had neither diabetes nor a prediabetic condition but were given the vinegar solution) also experienced a reduction in insulin levels in the blood. These findings are significant because, in addition to the nerve damage caused by perpetually elevated blood sugar levels, several chronic conditions, including heart disease, have been linked to excess insulin in the blood over prolonged periods of time.

More studies certainly need to be done to confirm the extent of vinegar's benefits for type 2 diabetes patients and those at risk of developing this increasingly common disease. But for now, people with type 2 diabetes might be wise to talk with their doctors or dietitians about consuming more vinegar.

MAKING A HEALTHY DIET EASIER TO SWALLOW

Some of our strongest natural weapons against cancer and aging are fruits and vegetables. The antioxidants and phytochemicals they contain seem to hold real promise in lowering our risk of many types of cancer. Their antioxidants also help to protect cells from the free-radical damage that is thought to underlie many of the changes we associate with aging. Protected cells don't wear out and need replacing as often as cells that aren't bathed in antioxidants. Scientists think this continual cell replacement may be at the root of aging.

The U.S. government's 2005 Dietary Guidelines recommend that the average person eat about two cups of fruit and two- and-a-half cups of vegetables every day. One way to add excitement and variety to all those vegetables is to use vinegar liberally as a seasoning.

- Rice vinegar and a little soy sauce give veggies an Asian flavor or can form the base of an Asian coleslaw.

- Red wine vinegar or white wine vinegar can turn boring vegetables into a quick-and-easy marinated-vegetable salad that's ready to grab out of the refrigerator whenever hunger strikes. Just chop your favorite veggies, put them in a bowl with a marinade of vinegar, herbs, and a dash of olive oil, and let them sit for at least an hour. (You don't need much oil to make the marinade stick to the veggies, so go light, and be sure you choose olive oil.)

- Toss chopped vegetables in a vinegar-and-olive-oil salad dressing before loading them on skewers and putting them on the backyard grill. The aroma and flavor will actually have your family asking for seconds.

- After steaming vegetables, drizzle a little of your favorite vinegar over them instead of adding butter or salt. They'll taste so good, you may never get to the meat on your plate.

By enhancing the flavor of vegetables with vinegar, you and your family will be inclined to eat more of them. And that—many researchers and doctors would agree—will likely go a long way toward protecting your body's cells from the damage that can lead to cancer and other problems of aging.

Vinegar can also help you have your dessert and cut calories, too. Use a splash of balsamic vinegar to bring out the sweetness and flavor of strawberries without any added sugar. Try it on other fruits that you might sprinkle sugar on—you'll be pleasantly surprised at the difference a bit of balsamic vinegar can make. And for a real unexpected treat on a hot summer evening, drizzle balsamic vinegar—instead of high-fat, sugary caramel or chocolate sauce—on a dish of reduced-fat vanilla ice cream. Can't imagine that combination? Just try it.

REMOVING HARMFUL SUBSTANCES FROM PRODUCE

Some people are concerned that eating large amounts of fruits and vegetables may lead to an unhealthy consumption of pesticides and other farm-chemical residues. Vinegar can lend a hand here, too. Washing produce in a mixture of water and vinegar appears to help remove certain pesticides, according to the small amount of research that has been published. Vinegar also appears to be helpful in getting rid of harmful bacteria on fruits and vegetables.

To help remove potentially harmful residues, mix a solution of 10 percent vinegar to 90 percent water (for example, mix one cup of white vinegar in nine cups of water). Then, place the produce in the vinegar solution, let it soak briefly, and then swish it around in the solution. Finally, rinse the produce thoroughly. Do not use this process on tender, fragile fruits, such as berries, that might be damaged in the process or soak up too much vinegar through their porous skins.

REMEDIES FOR MINOR AILMENTS

Vinegar's potential for treating or preventing major medical problems is of interest to almost everyone. But it also has been cherished as a home remedy for some common minor ailments for centuries. Although they're not life-or-death issues, these minor health problems can be uncomfortable, and there is often little modern medicine can offer in the way of a cure. So you may want to give vinegar a shot to determine for yourself if it can help.

(Remember, it's always best when trying any remedy for the first time to run it past your doctor to be sure there is no reason you should not try it.)

Stomach upset: To settle minor stomach upset, try a simple cider vinegar tonic with a meal. Drinking a mixture of a spoonful of vinegar in a glass of water is said to improve digestion and ease minor stomach upset by stimulating digestive juices.

Common cold symptoms: Apple cider vinegar is also an age-old treatment for symptoms of the common cold. For a sore throat, mix one teaspoon of apple cider vinegar into a glass of water; gargle with a mouthful of the solution and then swallow it, repeating until you've finished all the solution in the glass. For a natural cough syrup, mix half a tablespoon apple cider vinegar with half a tablespoon honey and swallow. Finally, you can add a quarter-cup of apple cider vinegar to the recommended amount of water in your room vaporizer to help with congestion.

Itching or stinging from minor insect bites: In the folklore of New England, rural Indiana, and parts of the Southwest, a vinegar wash is sometimes used for treating bites and stings. (However, if the person bitten has a known allergy to insect venom or begins to exhibit signs of a serious allergic reaction, such as widespread hives, swelling of the face or mouth, difficulty breathing, or loss of consciousness, skip the home remedies and seek immediate medical attention.) Pour undiluted vinegar over the bite or sting, avoiding surrounding healthy skin as much as possible.

Athlete's foot: One way to eliminate athlete's foot (or other fungal infection) is to create an environment that is inhospitable to the fungus that causes the condition. The Amish traditionally use a footbath of vinegar and water to discourage the growth of athlete's foot fungus. To try this remedy, mix one cup of vinegar into two quarts of water in a basin or pan. Soak your feet in this solution every night for 15 to 30 minutes, using a fresh solution each night. Or, if you prefer, mix up a solution using one cup of vinegar and one cup of water. Apply the solution to the affected parts of your feet with a cotton ball. Let your feet dry completely before putting on socks and/or shoes.

OLIVE OIL: PERENNIAL HEALTH FOOD

A diet that is rich in olive oil has enhanced the health of people living in the Mediterranean region for thousands of years. Within the past century, however, olive oil's benefits have also been scientifically investigated, acknowledged, and proclaimed across the globe.

Historians believe olive use spread throughout the rest of the Mediterranean region about 6,000 years ago. Phoenicians carried olive trees to what is now southern Europe, as well as to Egypt and other areas along the North African coast. Like garlic, olive remnants have been found inside Egyptian tombs, signifying the important role they played in that culture.

Later, the Greeks and Romans put olives to good use. People in both of these ancient civilizations used olive oil to counteract poisons and to treat open wounds, insect bites, headaches, and stomach and digestive problems. They also applied olive oil to the body before bathing (it functioned as soap) and then again afterward to moisturize the skin and to form a barrier against dirt and the sun's rays. The Romans took olives along in their travels, planting them wherever they went and spreading their beneficial qualities to many regions.

HEALING THROUGH THE AGES

As the olive migrated, folk remedies that used olive oil evolved to reflect the times and maladies of different regions. Olive oil was taken by mouth, spread on the skin, and dropped into the ears or nose. People considered it both a cure and a preventative measure for many afflictions. Here are some popular folk remedies that have been used over the years:

- Take a spoonful or two to treat an upset stomach, difficult digestion, or constipation or to reduce the body's absorption of alcohol from alcoholic beverages.
- Apply to skin to prevent dryness and wrinkles, to soften the skin, and to treat acne.
- Use on the hair to make it shiny and to treat dandruff.
- Strengthen nails by soaking them in warm olive oil.

- Ease aching muscles by massaging them with olive oil.
- Lower blood pressure by boiling olive tree leaves and drinking the "tea."
- Clear nasal congestion with drops of olive oil in the nose.

Chronic diseases and conditions that are caused, in part, by unhealthy foods and sedentary lifestyles plague many societies today. The good news is olive oil may help with the worst of them, including heart disease, hypertension (high blood pressure), metabolic syndrome, inflammation, cancer, diabetes, and problems associated with obesity.

These conditions take many years to develop, but inactivity and consumption of too much solid fat (saturated fat and trans fat) greatly increase your chances of having to deal with them. However, olive oil and diets rich in monounsaturated fat may help combat the development of some chronic conditions.

FAT FACTS

It may seem remarkable that such a small dietary change—switching from one type of fat to another—can significantly impact your health, but the type of fat you fancy really matters. Some fats, especially olive oil, have more healthful properties than others, so to make the right choices, it's important to know the differences among the various kinds. Let's review the four types of dietary fats, also known as fatty acids.

Monounsaturated fat. This is the healthiest type of fat. It promotes heart health and might help prevent cancer and a host of other ailments. Monounsaturated fat helps lower "bad" LDL cholesterol levels without negatively affecting the "good" HDL cholesterol. Olive oil, peanut oil, canola oil, and avocados are rich in healthy monounsaturated fat.

Polyunsaturated fat. Polyunsaturated fat is moderately healthy. It lowers LDL cholesterol, which is good, but it also reduces levels of artery-clearing HDL cholesterol. Polyunsaturated fat is usually liquid at room temperature and is the predominant type of fatty acid in soybean oil, safflower oil, corn oil, and several other vegetable oils.

Saturated fat. This fat is unhealthy because the body turns it into artery-clogging cholesterol, which is harmful to your heart. Saturated fat is mostly found in animal products and is solid at room temperature. It is the white fat you see along the edge or marbled throughout a piece of meat and is the fat in the skin of poultry. It is also "hidden" in whole milk and foods made from whole milk, as well as in tropical oils such as coconut oil. Dietitians recommend that people eat only small amounts of saturated fat.

Trans fat. Trans fat is the worst type of fat; you're best off avoiding it. Most trans fat is manufactured by forcing hydrogen into liquid polyunsaturated fat in a process called hydrogenation. The process can create a solid fat product—margarine is made this way. Hydrogenation gives foods that contain trans fats a longer shelf life and helps stabilize their flavors, but your body pays a big price.

A WORD OF CAUTION

Using olive oil as a folk remedy may not be safe for children. In November 2005, an article in *Archives of Pediatrics & Adolescent Medicine* and an ensuing report by Reuters Health cautioned caregivers against giving infants and young children a dose of olive oil to treat digestive problems, fussiness, and stuffy noses. Oil administered through the mouth or nose may be inhaled into the lungs and can cause lipoid pneumonia. You should always consult a pediatrician before trying any treatment—whether folk remedy or over-the-counter drug—on a child.

AN OLIVE'S OMEGAS

There are two important polyunsaturated fats that are essential for human health, but the body cannot make them. This means we must get them from the foods we eat. These two essential fatty acids are alpha-linolenic acid, an omega-3 fatty acid, and linoleic acid, an omega-6 fatty acid. The body gets both from olive oil. Omega-3 oils are the healthiest. They are part of a group of substances called prostaglandins that help keep blood cells from sticking together, increase blood flow, and reduce inflammation. This makes omega-3 oils useful in preventing cardiovascular disease as well as inflammatory conditions, such as arthritis.

Omega-6 oils are healthy, too, but they are not quite as helpful as omega-3's. Omega-6's can help form prostaglandins that are similarly beneficial to the ones produced by omega-3's, but they can also produce harmful prostaglandins. The unfavorable prostaglandins increase blood-cell stickiness and promote cardiovascular disease, and they also appear to be linked to the formation of cancer. To encourage your body to make beneficial prostaglandins from omega-6 oils, you should decrease the amount of animal fats you eat. Too many animal fats tend to push your body into using omega-6 oils to make the unfavorable prostaglandins rather than the helpful ones.

The research is inconclusive about how much omega-6 you should eat compared to the amount of omega-3. Many researchers suggest consuming one to four times more omega-6's than omega-3's. However, the typical American eats anywhere from 11 to 30 times more omega-6's than omega-3's.

The U.S. Dietary Reference Intakes for essential fatty acids recommends the consumption of omega-6 and omega-3 fats in a ratio of 10-to-1. This means consuming ten times more omega-6's than omega-3's. Lucky for us, nature provided that exact ratio of fat in each little olive. The linoleic-to-linolenic ratio is about 10-to-1.

GET HEART HELP
FROM OLIVE OIL

Research abounds regarding the benefits of monounsaturated fat. Other studies are showing that the potent phytochemicals (those substances in plants that may have health benefits for people) in olive oil—specifically, a group called phenolic compounds—appear to promote good health.

Studies have shown that a phytochemical in olive oil called hydroxytyrosol "thins" the blood. Other phytochemicals reduce inflammation of the blood vessels, prevent oxidation of fats in the bloodstream, protect blood vessel walls, and dilate the blood vessels for improved circulation.

CHOLESTEROL COMBATANT

Olive oil boosts heart health by keeping a lid on cholesterol levels. It lowers total cholesterol, LDL cholesterol, and triglyceride levels. Some studies show that it does not affect HDL cholesterol; others show that it slightly increases HDL levels. A 2002 article in *The American Journal of Medicine* reported that total cholesterol levels decrease an average of 13.4 percent and LDL cholesterol levels drop an average of 18 percent when people replace saturated fat with monounsaturated fat in their diets. These results seem to hold for middle-aged and older adults who have high blood cholesterol levels.

The polyphenolic compounds (types of phytochemicals) in olive oil appear to play a big part in protecting blood vessels. Three polyphenols, oleuropein, tyrosol, and hydroxytyrosol, are believed to be particularly helpful. Numerous studies have shown that polyphenols and monounsaturated fat help keep LDL cholesterol from being oxidized and getting stuck to the inner walls of arteries, which forms the plaque that hampers blood flow.

Polyphenolic compounds are also responsible for protecting two enzymes—glutathione reductase and glutathione peroxidase—that fight free radicals in the body. Without these enzymes, free radicals can damage healthy cells, potentially leading to cancer and other serious health problems.

THE MEDITERRANEAN DIET

The Mediterranean diet (one that is high in monounsaturated fat from olive oil and moderate in calories) made headlines when an Italian study appeared in the *Journal of the American Medical Association* in September 2004. The study followed two groups of 90 people who had metabolic syndrome (see sidebar) for two years. During the study, both groups increased their activity levels by 60 percent.

One study group was given detailed instructions about how to increase the whole grains, vegetables, fruits, nuts, and olive oil in their diets. The other 90 subjects consumed a "control" diet (50 percent to 60 percent of calories from carbohydrates, 15 percent to 20 percent of calories from protein, and less than 30 percent of calories from fat). After two years, those on the Mediterranean diet showed improvement in cholesterol levels, significantly less C-reactive protein in their blood, less insulin resistance, more weight loss, and improvements in the condition of their blood-vessel walls. A follow-up study two years later revealed only 40 of the original 90 people on the Mediterranean diet still had metabolic syndrome, compared with 78 people in the control group.

MORE HEARTFELT EVIDENCE

A French study published in the *International Journal of Obesity-Related Metabolic Disorders* in June 2003 added to the evidence in favor of olive oil as a heart helper. Thirty-two people ate either a high-carbohydrate diet or one that was high in monounsaturated fat. After eight weeks, the people who consumed lots of mono-unsaturated fats had better triglyceride levels than those participants who were on the diet high in carbohydrates. Those who ate more monounsaturated fat also had less oxidative stress, a condition in which there are more free radicals than the body can

Metabolic syndrome is a cluster of conditions that increases the risk of coronary artery disease and type 2 diabetes. In general, if a person has three or more of the conditions listed below, he or she likely has metabolic syndrome (which is sometimes called insulin resistance syndrome).

- Excess weight, especially in the abdominal area
- High LDL cholesterol, low HDL cholesterol, and high triglyceride levels
- High blood pressure
- Insulin resistance (the body doesn't respond to insulin appropriately)
- "Thick" blood that is prone to clumping and clotting (as indicated by high levels of a substance called plasminogen activator inhibitor-1 in the blood)
- Inflamed blood vessels (as indicated by high levels in the blood of a compound named C-reactive protein)

handle and/or low levels of antioxidants. This condition puts the arteries at risk of damage and encourages heart disease (among other unhealthy effects). The diet rich in monounsaturated fat also appeared to protect against smooth-muscle-cell proliferation, another risk factor for atherosclerosis.

A BOON TO BLOOD PRESSURE

An Italian study published in the December 2003 issue of the *Journal of Hypertension* reviewed numerous research projects that looked at various factors that affect blood pressure. The review indicated that unsaturated fat reduced blood pressure. The researchers went on to say that olive oil in particular was uniquely able to reduce high blood pressure—much more than sunflower oil.

A large study that appeared a year later in *The American Journal of Clinical Nutrition* looked at the diets of more than 20,000 Greeks who did not have high blood pressure when the study began. The study found that those who ate the typical Mediterranean diet had lower blood pressure. Furthermore, when the effects of olive oil consumption were compared to those of vegetable oil consumption, olive oil was shown to have a more positive impact on blood pressure.

Spain is another country where olive oil is a staple in many households. People there typically use olive oil, sunflower oil (a mostly polyunsaturated oil), or a mixture of the two. Researchers in one Spanish study wanted to learn the role each of these oils played in blood pressure, as well as how the oils held up to cultural cooking methods in which oil is heated to a high temperature for frying and later reused several times.

The study, which was published in the December 2003 issue of *The American Journal of Clinical Nutrition,* examined samples of cooking oil from the kitchens of 538 study participants. Researchers measured the blood pressure and conducted blood tests on those participants and nearly 500 more "control" subjects. Here's what they found:

- Olive oil was resistant to heat degradation.
- Mixed oil and sunflower oil degraded more than olive oil alone when heated and reused.
- Those who used sunflower oil, whether or not it had deteriorated, had higher blood pressure levels than those who used olive oil.
- The higher the monounsaturated fat consumption, the lower the blood pressure tended to be.

At the end of the study, the researchers concluded that because olive oil does a better job of maintaining its healthful properties and because it positively influences blood cholesterol and blood pressure levels, it should be the oil of choice in everyone's kitchen.

COOLING INFLAMMATION

Inflammation within the body may occur in response to cigarette smoking or eating large amounts of saturated fat and trans fat. In overweight or obese people, excess fat from fat cells can float through the bloodstream and cause inflammation. Although inflammation can help the body, it can also hurt.

Certain dietary fats cause more of an inflammatory response than others. Trans fat and the saturated fat in animal foods stimulate inflammation. To a smaller extent, polyunsaturated fat in foods such as safflower oil, sunflower oil, and corn oil trigger inflammation, as well.

Again, this is where olive oil helps. Olive oil's phytonutrients—in this case phenolic compounds called squalene, beta-sitosterol, and tyrosol—don't cause the inflammation that other fats do.

WHAT IS INFLAMMATION?

Inflammation is the immune system's first line of defense against injury and infection. When an injury occurs, such as a simple cut on the finger, a set of events takes place within your body that forms a blood clot, fights infection, and begins the healing process. Inflammation is painful because blood vessels dilate upstream of the injury to bring more blood and nutrients to the injured area, but they constrict at the injury site. These actions result in fluids from the bloodstream pooling in tissue around the injury, which causes swelling and pressure that stimulate nerves and cause pain.

When inflammation continues unabated for long periods of time, damage can occur in organs, such as the colon, or in blood vessels. Indeed, chronic inflammation within the body is looking more and more like a serious contributor to cardiovascular (heart and blood vessel) disease. Inflammation may damage the inner lining of blood vessels, which encourages plaque deposits to form.

Scientists have discovered that inflammation can be reduced with low daily doses of aspirin or other nonsteroidal anti-inflammatory drugs (NSAIDs), which in turn appear to reduce the risk of diseases caused by inflammation. Fortunately, not only does olive oil not prompt the kind of inflammation other types of fat can, it actually has some ability to *reduce* inflammation, thanks to those helpful phytochemicals (squalene, beta-sitosterol, and tyrosol). So consuming olive oil on a regular basis may help decrease the risk of conditions linked to inflammation.

Yet another condition that appears to be linked to inflammation is type 2 diabetes, the most common form of diabetes that affects an estimated 20 million Americans. Having excess body fat seems to increase inflammation. As inflammation increases, so does insulin resistance. As insulin resistance increases, blood glucose levels rise and the risk of type 2 diabetes skyrockets.

WHAT IS OLEOCANTHAL AND HOW CAN IT HELP YOU?

An article published by Philadelphia researchers in the September 2005 issue of *Nature* identified a compound in olive oil called oleocanthal that has anti-inflammatory action. Their studies revealed that this compound can act like ibuprofen and other anti-inflammatory medications.

Olive oils differ widely in the amount of oleocanthal they possess. To get an idea of how oleocanthal-rich your olive oil of choice is, researchers suggest taking a sip of the oil to "see how strongly it stings the back of the throat." The stronger the sting, the more oleocanthal the oil contains. Fifty grams (nearly a quarter of a cup of olive oil) provides the same amount of anti-inflammatory action as 10 percent of the standard adult dose of ibuprofen.

Obviously, eating enough olive oil to equal a whole dose of ibuprofen is not a practical way to decrease your inflammation and pain. But consuming a moderate amount of olive oil daily—in place of most of the other fat you typically consume—over the long term may lessen chronic inflammation throughout the body and bloodstream. It might even somewhat diminish asthma and rheumatoid arthritis symptoms.

Future research will probably tell us more about olive oil's function in battling oxidation, inflammation, and all the multiple diseases and health conditions associated with them.

OLIVE OIL'S POSSIBLE ROLE IN CANCER PREVENTION

Many medical researchers believe cancers of the colon, prostate, and breast are linked to dietary fat intake. Typically, high-fat diets were blamed, but research is beginning to suggest the more important factor may be the type of fat in the diet. In Spain, Italy, and Greece, where olive oil is used in most households, cancer incidence is much lower than in northern Europe and the United States, where olive oil use isn't as widespread.

There is plenty of controversy regarding whether olive oil can play any part in helping to prevent breast cancer, but women who follow a

Mediterranean-style diet appear to have a lower risk of the disease. A study published in the March 2005 issue of the *Annals of Oncology* showed that oleic acid, the principal monounsaturated fat in olive oil, dramatically decreased the growth of aggressive forms of breast tumors in test tubes. When oleic acid was combined with the commonly used breast cancer drug Herceptin, the effectiveness of the drug was vastly improved.

Clearly, more studies are needed to determine olive oil's real relationship to cancer. In the meantime, moderation may be the key to reaping the benefits of olive oil without increasing risk.

DIABETES AND OLIVE OIL

People living with diabetes have to work hard to keep their blood sugar, also called blood glucose, levels under control. One way to do so is to eat a diet low in carbohydrates. Because people with diabetes are also at risk of developing heart disease, they are advised to limit their intake of dietary fat. Lately, researchers have been debating the best type of eating pattern for people with diabetes. Some research now indicates that a diet high in monounsaturated fat may be better than a low-fat, low-carbohydrate diet. Numerous studies have suggested that people with diabetes who consume a diet high in monounsaturated fat have the same level of control over blood sugar levels as those who eat a low-fat diabetic diet. But monounsaturated fat also helps keep triglyceride levels in check, reduce LDL cholesterol levels, and increase HDL cholesterol levels.

Researchers in Spain published an article in *The American Journal of Clinical Nutrition* in September 2003 that concluded calorie-controlled diabetic diets high in monounsaturated fat do not cause weight gain and are more pleasing to eat than low-fat diets. The researchers determined that a diet high in monounsaturated fat is a good idea for people with diabetes.

Research is still inconsistent as to whether monounsaturated fat actually plays a role in stabilizing blood glucose levels, but evidence is leaning that way. A review of a number of studies, which was done by German researchers and appeared in the journal of the German Diabetes Association, found that blood glucose levels were lower in people who ate a diet rich in monounsaturated fat than in people who ate a low-fat diet. Further, they said increasing monounsaturated-fat intake lowered LDL cholesterol levels in some, though not all, subjects.

WEIGHTY ISSUES

Medical professionals are greatly concerned about the obesity problem in the United States. Obesity often comes hand-in-hand with high levels of cholesterol and lipids in the blood, heart disease, high blood pressure, diabetes, certain cancers, and a higher rate of premature death.

Health-care professionals often recommend following a strict but healthy diet in order to lose weight. But there may be some good news for those over-weight folks who struggle to limit dietary fat. Research suggests that replac-ing other types of fats with monounsaturated fat, especially olive oil, helps people lose a moderate amount of weight without additional food restriction or physical activity. So just imagine what adding a lower-calorie diet and increased physical activity (which is always a good idea) to the consumption of monounsaturated fats like olive oil could do for your weight-loss efforts.

FDA scientists reviewed many different studies when they evaluated whether to allow health claims for monounsaturated fat on food labels in 2003. The researchers wanted to ensure that a proposed recommendation to eat 13.5 grams (one tablespoon) of olive oil per day wouldn't contribute to weight gain in the American population. A number of studies showed that when people substituted monounsaturated-fat-rich olive oil for saturated fat, they either maintained their weight or lost weight.

A diet high in monounsaturated fat and low in carbohydrates actually resulted in more weight loss than a low-fat, high-carbohydrate diet.

What's more, the FDA determined that eating 13.5 grams of monounsaturated fat in a dietary pattern low in saturated fat and cholesterol would reduce total blood cholesterol and LDL cholesterol levels by an average of 5 percent, result-ing in a 10 percent decrease in coronary heart disease. However, the FDA did not approve this particular claim for food labels. Instead, the agency approved a stronger claim linking the consumption of 23 grams (about two tablespoons) of olive oil to a decreased risk of coronary heart disease.

Another study showed that when people ate monounsaturated fat, they ate less. For example, when served bread with olive oil, participants ate 23 percent less bread than when they ate it with butter, a saturated fat. Scientists speculate that because monounsaturated fat is more satisfying than other types of fat, people eat less of it. Additionally, the body's metabolism of monounsaturated fat after a meal appears to be different from the metabolism of saturated fat. This difference in metabolism may be what causes slight weight loss. (Re-searchers haven't yet determined exactly how this works.)

Several other studies indicate that monounsaturated fat may even enhance the body's breakdown of stored fat. A study of rats that was published in the *British Journal of Nutrition* in December 2003 found that monounsaturated fat facilitated the release of fat from rats' fat cells. Also, insulin became less able to prevent the breakdown of fat, which made it easier for fat cells to release their stored fat for elimination by the body. Thus, an increase in monounsaturated fat in the diet (along with, presumably, an equivalent decrease in saturated-fat intake) may help with weight loss; results were opposite in the rats that were given polyunsaturated fat.

OH, THOSE POWERFUL OLIVES

Not all olives are created equal. Just as some varieties of apples are sweeter or more tart than others, different varieties of olives yield varying amounts of oil. Large black olives typically purchased in a can from the grocer's shelf may contain as little as 7 percent oil. These are table olives. At the other end of the spectrum, some olives contain up to 35 percent oil. These are the ones used for pressing.

Hundreds of olive varieties exist, but only several dozen are grown commercially around the world. Some varieties are bursting with health-promoting polyphenols, while others contain few. The type of olive used to make any particular bottle of oil is rarely listed on the label. However, for those labels that do have the information, the following table, which shows which olives are richest in beneficial polyphenols, will be helpful.

POLYPHENOL CONTENT OF SELECTED OLIVE VARIETIES

Very High	*High*	*Medium High*
Coratina	Bosana	Frantoio
Cornicabra	Chemlali	
Koroneiki	Manzanillo	
Moraiolo	Picholine	
Picual	Picholine marocaine	
	Verdial de huevar	

The time at which olives are harvested also plays a major role in flavor and polyphenol content. The peak time is a short period right as the olives ripen. Olives are at their prime for only about two or three weeks. Healthy compounds then rapidly diminish over the next two to five weeks.

WHAT COLORS SAY

Olive oils made from unripe, green olives have a light- to deep-green color. Oils made from ripe olives tend to be a golden- or light-yellow color. The color of olive oil is not an indicator of quality in relationship to culinary uses; however, if you're looking to get the most polyphenols from your olive oil, choose one with golden or yellow tints because they come from ripe olives and may contain more healing compounds.

LABEL LINGO

Here are some terms you might see on olive oil labels that describe extraction methods. The first two are cold extraction processes. Olive oils processed by these methods retain the vitamins, health-boosting phytochemicals, color, flavor, and aroma of the olives. The second two are heat-extraction processes. The heat used in these techniques takes a toll on olive oil. Excessive heat destroys many of the fragile nutrients and phytochemicals and just about all of the color, flavor, and aroma.

Cold pressed. This method removes the oil from olives through pressing and grinding. For the oil to be labeled "cold pressed," the heat generated by friction from the grinding must not exceed 86 degrees Fahrenheit. (Other oils, such as safflower and canola, are sometimes cold pressed, but for those oils, friction temperatures of up to 120 degrees Fahrenheit are allowed.)

Vacuum extraction. This is a cold-extraction method done in the absence of air and light at temperatures as low as 70 degrees Fahrenheit. Olives are crushed and ground, then mixed with water and churned in a device that uses a vacuum. The process ensures no air is introduced into the system and preserves the antioxidants and nutrients.

Expeller pressed. This method also uses grinding and pressing, but with extreme amounts of pressure, sometimes up to 15 tons per square inch. This intense amount of pressure creates a lot of heat and friction that takes the oil to temperatures of up to 300 degrees Fahrenheit.

Solvent extraction. This technique uses chemicals, such as hexane, to remove oil from olives. The oil is then boiled to get rid of the chemicals. The oil may then undergo additional heat processing, bleaching, or deodorizing, which leads to a bland oil, but one with a high smoke point and long shelf life.

OLIVE OIL OPTIONS

Rich, beautiful, and fragrant, olive oil is much like wine—taste is a matter of personal preference. The many variables that go into the production of olive oil yield dramatic differences in color, aroma, and flavor. The following factors impact the taste of olive oil:

- Variety of olive used
- Location and soil conditions where the olives were grown
- Environmental factors and weather during the growing season
- Olive ripeness
- Timing of the harvest
- Harvesting method
- Length of time between the harvest and pressing
- Pressing technique
- Packaging and storage methods

FREE ACIDS ARE BAD ACIDS

An olive oil's quality is determined by the amount of acidity, or free oleic acid, is contained in the oil. Higher-quality oils have lower acidity levels.

Wait, didn't we say that oleic acid has beneficial health properties? Yes, it does, but it is *free* oleic acid (a type of fatty acid) that indicates lesser quality. Oleic acid can either roam around by itself as a single fatty acid or it can be attached to other fat components.

To understand what this means, picture a capital letter "E." The vertical line of the "E" is the backbone—a triglyceride that is a common type of fat. Each of the three horizontal arms of the "E" contains a fatty acid, one or more of them being oleic acid. In this form, attached to the triglyceride, oleic acid is valuable. But if the oleic acid arm of the "E" triglyceride breaks off, it becomes free, or unbound, and is therefore called "free oleic acid."

Difficult growing conditions; olives picked too soon or too late; infestations of pests, such as olive flies; fungal diseases; damage or bruising during harvesting; and poor storage conditions all allow free oleic acid to form. When this happens, the oil begins to break down, diminishing its quality.

WHERE IN THE WORLD?

When buying olive oil, you'll see varieties from all over the globe. Most of the world's supply is produced from olives grown in Spain, Italy, and Greece, but other areas, including France and California, are in on the fun, too. Here's what you need to know about olive oil and geography:

- Spanish olive oil is typically golden yellow with a fruity, nutty flavor. Spain produces about 45 percent of the world's olive supply.

- Italian olive oil is often dark green and has an herbal aroma and a grassy flavor. Italy grows about 20 percent of the world's olives.

- Greek olive oil packs a strong flavor and aroma and tends to be green. Greece produces about 13 percent of the world's olive supply.

- French olive oil is typically pale in color and has a milder flavor than other varieties.

- Californian olive oil is light in color and flavor, with a bit of a fruity taste. Olives from different countries are often blended together to produce an oil variety. Or, olives from diverse areas of one country may be combined. These bulk-blended oils are the most economical but are still high quality. On the other hand, some producers only use olives that are grown in a specific area of a country. These regional oils are usually known for their unique flavors.

Estate olive oils are the cream of the crop. Estate oils are produced using olives from a single olive farm. These olives are usually handpicked, then pressed and bottled right at the estate. Expect to get the best flavor out of these varieties, but also expect to pay more.

MAKING THE GRADES

There are three basic grades of edible olive oil, and several types within each grade. Extra virgin includes "premium extra virgin" and "extra virgin"; virgin comprises "fine virgin," "virgin," and "semi-fine virgin"; and olive oil includes what used to be called "pure olive oil" and "refined oil."

All types of extra virgin and virgin oils are made from the first pressing of the olives, which removes about 90 percent of the olives' juice. Chemicals and high heat are not allowed in the production of extra virgin or virgin oils—no further processing or refining occurs after the pressing process. Neither extra virgin nor virgin oils are allowed to contain any refined olive oil.

At the head of the olive oil class sit the extra virgins, followed closely by the virgins. The difference between two oils and where they rank in the following hierarchy may be just half a percentage point of acidity. However, that is all it takes to distinguish between a very good oil and a great oil.

"Premium extra virgin olive oil" is nature's finest, thanks to its extremely low acidity (possibly as low as 0.225 percent). It is best suited for using uncooked in dishes where you can appreciate its exquisite aroma and flavor. Try it in salads, as a dip for bread, or as a condiment.

"Extra virgin olive oil" has a fruity taste and may be pale yellow to bright green in color. In general, the deeper the color, the more flavor it yields. IOOC regulations say extra virgin olive oil must have a superior flavor and contain no more than 0.8 percent acidity, but other regulators set the acidity cut-off point at 1 percent. As with the premium version, it is best to use extra virgin olive oil uncooked in order to appreciate its flavor.

"Fine virgin olive oil" must have a "good" taste (as judged by IOOC standards) and an acidity level of no more than 1.5 percent. Fine virgin olive oil is less expensive than extra virgin oil but is close in quality and is good uncooked.

"Virgin olive oil" must have a "good" taste, and its acidity must be 2 percent or less. Like other virgin oils, it cannot contain any refined oil. Virgin olive oil is good for cooking, but it also has enough flavor to be enjoyed uncooked.

"Semi-fine virgin olive oil" must have an acidity no higher than 3.3 percent. It is good for cooking but doesn't have enough flavor to be enjoyed uncooked.

Some olive oil is further refined after the first pressing. These three types of oils can no longer bear the title "virgin."

COLOR CONSIDERATIONS

Green olive oils come from unripe olives and impart a slightly bitter, pungent flavor. Emerald-tinged oils have fruity, grassy, and peppery flavors that dominate the foods in which you use them. These oils are great with neutral-flavored foods that allow their bold flavors to shine. You can pair green olive oils with strongly flavored foods as long as they complement the oils' pungent tastes.

Olive oils that glimmer with a golden color are made from ripe olives. Olives turn from green to bluish-purple to black as they ripen. Oils made from ripe olives have a milder, smoother, somewhat buttery taste without bitterness. These oils are perfect for foods with subtle flavors because the gentle taste of a ripe olive oil won't overshadow mildly flavored foods.

OLDER ISN'T BETTER

Unlike wine, oil does not improve with age. As olive oil gets older, it gradually breaks down, more free oleic acid is formed, the acidity level rises, and flavor weakens. Extra-virgin oils keep better because they have a low acidity level to start with, but you should use lower-quality oils within months because they start out with higher acidity levels. As oil sits on your shelf, its acidity level rises daily, and soon it is not palatable. You'll get the best quality and flavor from your olive oil if you use it within a year of pressing. Olive oil remains at its peak for about two or three months after pressing, but unfortunately, few labels carry bottling dates or "use by" dates, let alone pressing dates.

More is at issue than flavor, however. Research shows the nutrients in olive oil degrade over time. In a study that appeared in the May 2004 issue of the *Journal of Agriculture and Food Chemistry,* Spanish researchers tested virgin olive oil that had been stored for 12 months under perfect conditions. What they found was quite surprising: After 12 months, many of the oil's prime healing substances had practically vanished. All the vitamin E was gone, as much as 30 percent of the chlorophyll had deteriorated, and 40 percent of the beta-carotene had disintegrated. Phenol levels had dropped dramatically, too.

And finally, when it comes to olive oil storage, the morals of the story are:

- If possible, determine the age of the olive oil you're buying, or buy from a store where product turnover is rapid.
- Store your olive oil in an airtight container in a dark place at room temperature. You can refrigerate or freeze most oils for long-term storage.
- Buy small amounts that you can use within a few months.

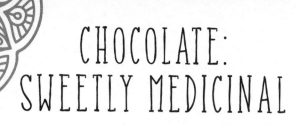

CHOCOLATE:
SWEETLY MEDICINAL

It's the very definition of good news: chocolate may be good for you!

Since ancient times, chocolate has been far more than a guilty pleasure. It has functioned as medicine, sacred ceremonial beverage, status symbol, even money. Chocolate comes from the seeds of the fruit of the cacao tree. The seemingly inedible, almond-size seeds, which are surrounded by sweet, tangy pulp, develop inside seed pods. The seed pods resemble footballs and grow out from the tree's trunk. The cacao tree is native to the tropical rain forests of Mesoamerica—the ancient region that covered the southern and eastern portions of Mexico, Guatemala, Belize, and parts of El Salvador and Honduras.

FLAVONOIDS: CACAO'S
ANTIOXIDANT SUPERSTARS

Researchers have discovered that cacao is rich in antioxidant phytochemicals, especially a type called polyphenols. Polyphenols are found not only in chocolate products but in fruits and fruit juices, vegetables, tea, coffee, red wine, and some grains and legumes. And the available research seems to strongly point to some role for polyphenols in preventing a variety of diseases.

The largest and most important class of polyphenols are the flavonoids. More than 5,000 flavonoids have been identified so far, and they have begun to attract a lot of attention for their potential health benefits. Among the flavonoid-rich foods that have shown promise lately are strawberries and blueberries, garlic, red wine, and tea. But these plant foods can't hold a candle to cacao-rich cocoa products when it comes to flavonoid content and antioxidant power. Cocoa, for example, has almost twice the antioxidants found in red wine and close to three times the antioxidants in green tea, when compared in equal amounts.

One of the flavonoids in cacao (known as cocoa flavonoids, or cocoa polyphenols) gaining a particular reputation for healing is epicatechin. One Harvard Medical School scientist is so impressed by epicatechin's effects that he has said it should be considered essential for human health and, therefore, raised to the status of a vitamin. He's also stated that the health benefits of epicatechin are so striking that it may rival penicillin and anesthesia in terms of importance to public health.

The researcher developed his views on epicatechin after spending years studying the health benefits of heavy cocoa drinking on an isolated tribe of people called the Kuna, who live on islands off the coast of Panama. The Kuna drink up to 40 cups of natural unsweetened cocoa per person every week. The scientist, working with an international team of colleagues, found that the island Kuna have remarkably low rates (less than 10 percent) of four of the five most common killer diseases in the industrialized world: heart disease, stroke, cancer, and diabetes. And the research further indicates that the Kuna's high intake of epicatechin from their cocoa is a primary cause of the low disease rates. Indeed, when tribe members leave their isolated islands to settle on mainland Panama—where they drink far less of the natural cocoa—their disease rates tend to go up.

In addition to demonstrating the healing potential of cocoa, the Kuna research highlights an important point about that potential. The Kuna not only drink large quantities of cocoa, the cocoa they drink has a very high flavonoid content—far higher than the flavonoid content of many of the sweetened, high-calorie, high-fat cocoa and chocolate products found on grocery-store shelves. And that's essential to its apparent health benefits. The Kuna grow their own cacao beans, gently roast and minimally process them, and use them to make an unadulterated cocoa that has a very high percentage of cocoa solids. And it's the cocoa solids that contain the flavonoids.

BOLD IS HEALTHY

Phytochemicals are often the substances responsible for the colors, aromas, and flavors of plants. So a bold appearance, strong taste, and/or pungent scent generally signals that a plant is rich in phytochemicals—and therefore loaded with antioxidant potential. When it comes to chocolate, the more of cacao's natural bitterness that remains in the product, the higher in phytochemicals (flavonoids) it tends to be.

Flavonoids, however, also give natural chocolate a very bitter taste. So in an effort to please their sweet-toothed consumers, chocolate manufacturers have traditionally tried to tame that natural bitterness by removing flavonoids and/or masking their taste. Nearly every step of the typical processes that turn cacao beans into chocolate and cocoa—including fermenting, roasting, and Dutching—removes some of the flavonoids. Likewise, adding ingredients such as sugar and milk to chocolate or cocoa—again, to mask or replace bitterness—leaves less room for cocoa solids and therefore results in a lower-flavonoid product.

While the rest of us can't control the way our cacao is grown and processed, as the Kuna do, we can increase our chances of getting and benefiting from cocoa flavonoids by opting for cocoa and chocolates with the most cocoa solids and the least sugar and milk added. You'll find advice on that later in the chapter. First, however, let's look at some of the studies that illustrate and support the specific disease-fighting effects of chocolate and cocoa.

COCOA FLAVONOIDS
AND DISEASE

In the past several years, scientists have produced some compelling research suggesting that cocoa flavonoids can help lower blood pressure, improve blood-vessel function, make blood less likely to form dangerous clots, and prevent the creation of artery-clogging blood-cholesterol molecules. All of these effects help ensure smooth, adequate, and uninterrupted blood flow to the heart and brain, lowering the risk of heart attack and stroke.

Blood Pressure. In a study published in August 2003 in the *Journal of the American Medical Association,* researchers discovered that eating dark chocolate helped individuals lower mild high blood pressure, while eating white chocolate did not provide the same benefits. The study included 13 men and women, ages 55 to 64, who had untreated mild high blood pressure. Each participant ate 90 grams of either dark chocolate or white chocolate each day for two weeks. Before the two-week experiment ended, those who ate the dark chocolate had significantly lower blood pressure, while the folks who ate white chocolate showed no such improvement. (Dark chocolate, you'll remember, contains chocolate liquor, made of cocoa solids and cocoa butter. White chocolate does not contain chocolate liquor and therefore provides no flavonoid-containing cocoa solids.)

In a similar study in Italy, published in 2005 in the journal *Hypertension,* researchers studied ten men and ten women who had high blood pressure. They were randomly assigned to eat either 100 grams of flavonoid-rich dark chocolate or 90 grams of flavonoid-free white chocolate each day for 15 days without increasing their total calorie intake (they were instructed to lower their calorie intake from other foods to compensate). Then, after a one-week break, they switched, with the subjects who previously ate dark chocolate daily now eating white chocolate, and vice versa, for another 15 days. The results: When the subjects ate dark chocolate, their systolic blood pressure (the upper number) dropped an average of 12 points and their diastolic pressure (the bottom number) dipped an average of 8. Eating white chocolate provided no such benefits.

A 2007 review of ten different studies of chocolate's effects on blood pressure indicated that flavonoid-rich cocoa and chocolate can indeed have a place in a blood-pressure lowering diet as long as the total calorie count of the diet stays the same. On average, chocolate products lowered systolic pressure by 4 to 5 points and diastolic by 2 to 3—enough to lower heart disease risk by 10 percent and stroke risk by 20 percent. The scientists did note, however, that because the studies were short term, it's unclear if the same effects would occur with consumption of small amounts of chocolate over the long term.

Blood Vessel Function. In studies that were published in the Journal of the *American College of Cardiology* in 2005 and in *Proceedings of the National Academy of Sciences* in 2006, researchers demonstrated that the flavonoids (specifically, epicatechin) in flavonoid-rich cocoa beverages trigger the production of a natural substance called nitric oxide. Nitric oxide, in turn, causes blood vessels to dilate (relax), allowing for smoother blood flow.

CHOCOLATE'S OTHER NUTRIENTS

Chocolate is also a good source of certain vitamins and minerals your body needs to stay healthy, including vitamins C, D, and E; B-complex vitamins; and the minerals iron, copper, phosphorus, zinc, calcium, and potassium. Cocoa is also the greatest natural source of magnesium, a deficiency of which is associated with high blood pressure, heart disease, diabetes, joint problems, and premenstrual syndrome.

Flavonoid-rich cocoa may even benefit the compromised blood-vessel function of smokers, to the point of potentially reversing some of the vessel damage caused by smoking, according to a study published in the *Journal of Cardiovascular Pharmacology* in March 2007. In smokers, the activity of endothelial cells (cells lining artery walls) is reduced; this reduction in activity is an early signal of blood-vessel diseases such as hardening of the arteries (atherosclerosis). In the two-part smoker study, 11 healthy male smokers first drank a series of specially made flavonoid-rich cocoa beverages containing 28 milligrams to 918 milligrams of flavonols (a subgroup of flavonoids). Two hours after they drank the beverage with 179 milligrams of flavonols, their blood-vessel function showed a 50 percent improvement. As they drank the cocoas with greater amounts of flavonols, the benefits increased. After they drank the cocoa with 918 milligrams, their cigarette-induced blood vessel damage appeared to have been reversed to the extent that their blood vessels functioned as well as those of someone with no risk factors for cardiovascular disease.

The first stage of the trial was followed by seven days of drinking three daily doses of the special cocoa (for a total of 918 milligrams of flavonols each day) to determine if the benefits continued. The subjects' blood flow improved each day, and after taking a 306-milligram dose on day seven, their cigarette-induced damage had nearly been reversed once again. The study paper indicated that the level of improvement in blood-vessel function after seven days of consuming the flavonol-rich cocoa was similar to the improvements produced by long-term treatment with statin drugs. (The researchers also noted that these improvements caused by cocoa flavonoids did not appear to be the result of their antioxidant effects.) One week after the end of the study, however, the subjects' blood-vessel function had returned to pre-study levels, indicating that cocoa drinking would have to continue to sustain these benefits. The authors also noted that larger studies need to be conducted to confirm these very exciting findings.

In another study released in March 2007, scientists found that consuming eight ounces of special flavonoid-rich cocoa every day for six weeks significantly improved the blood vessel health of people who were mildly obese. In the study, 45 mildly obese adults consumed either a flavonoid-rich, dark-chocolate cocoa mix sweetened with sugar; an artificially sweetened version of the same cocoa mix; or a placebo (control) mix made of sweetened whey powder. The artificially sweetened cocoa mix was associated with a 39 percent improvement in blood flow, and the sugared cocoa was linked with a 23 percent improvement. The placebo mix, however, *lowered* blood flow by 12 percent.

Blood Clotting. When the inner walls of arteries are narrowed by deposits of cholesterol and other debris, a blood clot can easily shut down the blood supply to the organ fed by the artery—leading to a heart attack, stroke, or other serious tissue damage. For that reason, many heart patients are prescribed a daily 81 milligram aspirin tablet, which thins their blood and helps prevent clots. In a 2002 study, scientists were astonished to find that drinking a flavonoid-rich cocoa drink could be just as effective as the aspirin at preventing clots. The research found similar reactions to both treatments in a group of 20- to 40-year-olds. Both the cocoa drink and the aspirin kept blood platelets from sticking together and forming clots. The researchers stopped short of suggesting that heart patients who have been prescribed a daily aspirin should drink cocoa instead. (And you should *NOT* stop taking any medication that has been prescribed for you without first consulting your doctor.) But for people at risk who can't take aspirin every day, it's possible that eating more flavonoid-rich foods could provide similar benefits.

Blood Cholesterol. Consuming saturated fat in food can increase total blood-cholesterol levels and, especially, levels of LDL cholesterol, the so-called "bad" form of blood cholesterol. Having too much LDL cholesterol is a risk factor for cardiovascular diseases, including heart attack and stroke, because LDL molecules tend to deposit excess cholesterol on the inner lining of artery walls, narrowing the arteries and setting the stage for a clot to cut off blood flow to the heart or brain. Scientists have discovered, however, that not all LDL molecules are equally damaging. It appears that LDL molecules that have been oxidized are the true culprits in clogging arteries. And that's where cocoa flavonoids may help. First, research suggests cocoa flavonoids may lower LDL levels. For example, in the 2005 study of Italians with high blood pressure, cited previously, the subjects who consumed flavonoid-rich dark chocolate experienced a 10 percent decrease in their LDL levels, in addition to a drop in blood pressure. Second, two 2001 studies showed that cocoa flavonoids can actually protect LDL molecules from oxidation.

In another bit of good news, scientists have determined that even the fat in cacao isn't so bad. Although cocoa butter is technically a saturated fat, it does not appear to increase LDL levels in the blood the way other saturated fats do. Half the saturated fat in cocoa butter is stearic acid, which studies indicate has a neutral effect on blood cholesterol.

Chocolate also contains some oleic acid—the same type of monounsaturated fat found in olive oil, which can actually help lower LDL levels and boost levels of high-density lipoproteins (HDLs)—the "good" form of cholesterol that helps remove excess cholesterol from the blood.

CANCER

Study after study has demonstrated that a high intake of fruits and vegetables is associated with a reduced risk of several common cancers, such as those of the lung, colon, prostate, and breast. Scientists suspect that the reduction in risk comes, at least in part, from the antioxidants in those plant foods. Further, several laboratory, animal, and human studies point specifically to flavonoids as providing protection against cancer-promoting free-radical damage. And of the plant-based beverages known to be rich in flavonoids, Cornell University food scientists were amazed to find that cocoa contains the highest levels by far.

There is even some early evidence suggesting cocoa flavonoids may help fight skin cancer. In 2006, German researchers reported on their study of 24 women who added cocoa to their breakfast every day for about three months. Half the women consumed a flavonoid-heavy hot cocoa, and the others drank a cocoa that had few flavonoids. At the end of the trial, the researchers applied UV light—like that given off by the sun and found to cause skin cancer—to each subject's skin. The skin of the women who drank the high-flavonoid cocoa did not redden as much as the skin of the women who drank the flavonoid-poor cocoa, suggesting the flavonoids prompted some type of innate skin protection.

MEMORY AND COGNITION

Cocoa flavonoids may act in more than one way to benefit mental performance, particularly in people with certain types of dementia. For example, free-radical damage and inflammation in the brain have both been cited as potential contributors to the memory problems and cognitive decline that can occur with age and that are characteristic of dementias. We've already explored the amazingly powerful antioxidant effects of cocoa flavonoids. But these flavonoids also appear to suppress leukotrienes (substances that trigger inflammation in the body) and increase forms of anti-inflammatory nitric oxide.

In addition, the improvement in the health and function of blood vessels and the increased circulation that appear to result from consuming cocoa flavonoids may prove beneficial for those suffering dementia or other problems related to poor blood flow to the brain. In British research that was reported at the February 2007 annual meeting of the American Association for the Advancement of Science, drinking a flavonoid-rich cocoa beverage increased blood flow to key areas of the brain for two to three hours following ingestion. This increase in blood flow to the brain, scientists speculate, may be the result of greater amounts of nitric oxide in the circulation prompted by the cocoa flavonoids.

Some scientists are now considering the prospect of using cocoa flavonoids to help people with dementia and those who have had a stroke, as well as to enhance brain function in people suffering from fatigue, sleep deprivation, or poor circulation to the brain due to the aging of blood vessels.

ENJOYING CHOCOLATE WISELY

With such promising evidence of chocolate's healing potential, why *isn't* it considered a health food? Despite the persistence of the myth, it's not because chocolate causes acne. It doesn't. (Although because we tend to reach for comfort foods when we're under stress, and stress *can* aggravate acne, it's an easy myth to believe.) And it's not because chocolate is especially dangerous to teeth. Like any other carbohydrate, chocolate can indeed serve as food for oral bacteria, which excrete the acids that eat away at tooth enamel. But because it has a smooth texture and literally melts in your mouth, chocolate is actually a little less likely to cause cavities than are, say, bread and other baked goods or candies such as licorice and caramel that tend to actually get stuck on or between teeth. As long as you practice good oral hygiene and brush, or at least rinse, after eating chocolate, it's not a major danger to your pearly whites.

No, the reason health experts aren't pushing chocolate as a health food is the high calorie counts of commonly consumed chocolate products. Chocolate is a relatively calorie-dense food to begin with, and the super-sweet, creamy, milky, high-fat versions so many Americans favor simply compound the problem. Such concentrated sources of calories could hardly be considered required eating in a nation battling overweight and obesity.

What's more, because so many folks find it so taste-tempting, there's a real concern that they'll find it difficult to moderate their consumption. The potential result is even more unwanted pounds. And those unwanted pounds would easily outweigh the health benefits described in this chapter. Overweight and obesity increase the risk of heart disease, stroke, diabetes, and some forms of cancer.

So, must you send chocolate, despite its healing powers, back to the forbidden-fruit category? No. As a matter of fact, making favorite foods totally off-limits can provoke feelings of deprivation that can trigger binging and other unhealthy eating habits, which can lead to the very weight gain you are trying to avoid. The better approach is to choose chocolate products that provide the most flavor and healing benefits for the fewest calories and then make room in your diet to accommodate them. It will take some effort—you'll need to check and compare labels to find the best calorie bargains—and self-discipline—you can't eat as much as you want without risking your health—but you'll be able to have your chocolate and keep your weight in check, too.

According to the government's Agricultural Research Service, when it comes to the common chocolate products that pack the most flavonoids and the greatest antioxidant punch, natural (rather than Dutched), unsweetened cocoa powders top the list. They also tend to be the lowest in calories and so can be the most weight-wise way to quench your chocolate desires. The process of Dutching, or alkalinizing, cocoa powder removes some of the natural flavonoids, so if you can find it, choose an un-Dutched dark-chocolate cocoa powder (not a milk-chocolate cocoa mix), and prepare it with water. Sugar-sweetened powders retain fewer flavonoids—the sugar leaves less room for flavonoid-containing cocoa solids—and, of course, are higher in calories, so try an unsweetened powder (if you can't handle it unsweetened, you'll at least be able to add only as much sugar as is absolutely necessary) or, if you can find one, an artificially sweetened one.

When it comes to solid chocolates, opt for dark chocolates. Milk chocolates typically have no more than half the amount of cocoa solids that dark chocolates contain—and therefore they have far fewer healing flavonoids and much less antioxidant power. With the added milk and sugar, milk chocolate bars simply have far less room for cocoa solids and are often considerably higher in empty calories (calories that provide no nutritional benefit other than energy). A typical milk chocolate bar contains 30 percent cacao, 20 percent milk solids, 1 percent vanilla and emulsifier, and *49 percent sugar.* Some research even suggests that milk may interfere with the absorption of the antioxidants in cacao. And don't even bother with white chocolate if you're looking for any health benefits. It contains only cocoa butter, not cocoa solids (so no healing flavonoids), and loads of sugar.

These days, it seems, there's been an explosion in varieties and brands of dark chocolates. So how do you choose? Again, you want the products that are highest in cocoa solids. A helpful clue to cocoa-solid content is the "% Cacao" that is being listed on more and more chocolates. It's not a guarantee of a hefty dose of cocoa solids, however. That's because the "% Cacao" refers not only to the cocoa solids but to the total percentage of ingredients that come from cacao beans, including cocoa powder and cocoa butter. But only the solids (including those within the cocoa powder) contain flavonoids. So even though two chocolate bars list "70% Cacao," for example, one can have fewer cocoa solids—and so fewer flavonoids—and more cocoa butter than the other. (The flavonoid content of a chocolate product may also be affected by such variables as the types of cacao beans used to create it, the soil and weather conditions those beans were grown in, the recipe and processing used, and the storage and handling of the finished product.) Still, in the absence of a label listing only the percentage of cocoa solids, it can be a helpful guide.

You'll also find useful information in the ingredients list and the Nutrition Facts panel. When comparing chocolates that have the same "% Cacao," look not only at the calorie counts but at which ingredients, other than those from cacao, have been added. Opt for the lowest-calorie product with the fewest non-cacao ingredients.

How much chocolate and/or cocoa is it okay to consume? Moderation is key. If natural cocoa, especially an unsweetened variety, satisfies your taste for chocolate, that's definitely the way to go. You can probably enjoy a few cups a day. Because of its calorie content, however, you shouldn't look to add solid chocolate regularly to your diet unless you really enjoy it. If you do, you'll need to make room for it in your diet and then enjoy only as much as you've made room for. That means that if you'd like to enjoy a square or two (but not much more) of cacao-rich dark chocolate every day, you'll need to cut back— by an equivalent number of calories or more—on other sugary or fatty foods you eat that day. (If you're also trying to lose weight, you'll need to cut back even further on other sources of empty calories and, preferably, increase your physical activity level, too.) Do not replace nutrient-rich foods, such as veg-etables, fruit, and whole grains, with chocolate. That would truly be shooting yourself in the foot. Instead, cut back on foods such as sugary, high-fat baked goods; ice cream; fatty dressings and sauces; salty, greasy fast foods and snack foods; sweetened sodas; and other types of candy.

Once you've made room in your daily diet, make time to truly enjoy your chocolate. Take a few moments, sit down, and slowly savor the deep, rich flavor and melt-in-your-mouth texture of a high-quality dark-chocolate square. And remind yourself that there's no need to feel guilty about satisfying your choco-late desires in a responsible, healthy way.

FROM THE
COMMON CUPBOARD

APRICOTS

Apricots are chock-full of beta-carotene and other carotenoids, the beautiful pigments that color fruits and vegetables. There are more than 400 different kinds and most, if not all, are antioxidants. Some of apricot's carotenoids such as lycopene, gamma carotene, and cryptoxanthin pack a much more powerful antioxidant punch than does beta-carotene, making them even more useful as cancer-fighters.

Apricots contain some vitamin C, which keeps skin and tissues supple and healthy. Vitamin C also has antioxidant properties and supports the immune system, helping the body make substances to fight off illnesses. Apricots are rich in fiber for their size, especially soluble fiber. This heart-healthy fiber lowers blood cholesterol levels and helps people with diabetes maintain stable blood sugar levels. You can count on apricots' insoluble fiber to keep the colon free of toxins and your bowels moving regularly.

Dried apricots, because they are concentrated, are a good source of iron. Three and a half ounces provide about 47 percent of the recommended dietary allowance for men and 31 percent for women.

BEETS AND BEET GREENS

Beets have long been valued for their rich flavor, sweet taste, and vital nutrients. Beets are particularly rich in the B vitamin folate, which is essential for preventing a certain type of anemia and birth defects that affect the spinal column. Folate may prevent cancer, too, by protecting the DNA in cells from damage and mutation. Mutated cells are often the beginning of cancerous cells. Beets contain a wealth of soluble and insoluble fiber—great for keeping the intestines toned.

Beet greens are packed with healing nutrients, including disease fighters such as vitamin A and potassium. Calcium, too, is available from this nutritional powerhouse. The variety of vitamins and minerals make these leafy greens an all-around heart-healthy vegetable.

If you are trying to quit smoking, beet greens may become your new friend. Just like soil, human blood has a pH value, and a slightly alkaline condition apparently triggers nicotine to stay in the blood longer, reducing the craving for more cigarettes. At the University of Nebraska Medical Center, researchers found that beet greens push blood pH slightly toward the alkaline side. Smokers who are trying to quit might try eating plenty of alkaline foods to reduce their need for nicotine. Other high-alkaline foods include dandelion greens, spinach, and raisins.

Beet greens are abundant in folate. This B vitamin protects lung cells from damage that can trigger cancer, so smokers get a double dose of prevention from these greens.

CABBAGE

Cabbage juice has been used to prevent and heal ulcers for more than 40 years. Current research at the Stanford University School of Medicine revealed that when ulcer patients drank 1 quart of raw cabbage juice each day, ulcers in the stomach and small intestine healed in about five days. People who ate cabbage instead of drinking the juice also had faster healing times than those who did not eat cabbage.

Cabbage accomplishes this by killing bacteria, including the ulcer-causing H. pylori. Secondly, it contains a phytochemical called gefarnate that coaxes stomach cells into making extra mucus, which protects the stomach wall from digestive acid.

As a cruciferous family member, cabbages of all types help fight the war on cancer. Two types of darker-colored cabbage—savoy and bok choy—also provide beta-carotene.

CARROTS

Modern science has determined that carrots do much more than help eyesight. They offer a natural defense against heart disease, strokes, cancer, cataracts, and even constipation. And it only takes one carrot a day to dramatically reduce health risks. Studies show that a humble carrot a day reduced the risk of heart attack in women by 22 percent, and a carrot a day five days per week reduced women's stroke risk by 68 percent. Women who did have a stroke were less likely to die or be disabled. Scientists believe that phytochemicals (plant chemicals) in carrots protect oxygen-deprived brain cells.

Lung cancer risk plunged by 60 percent in a different study when a carrot was eaten twice a week. The incidence of other cancers, such as stomach, mouth, and those of the female reproductive tract, are also decreased by eating carrots.

One raw carrot or 1/2 cup cooked carrots supplies two to three times the recommended daily intake of vitamin A in the form of protective beta-carotene.

Carrots contain other carotenoids that are even more potent cancer warriors than beta-carotene: alpha-carotene, gamma-carotene, lycopene, and lutein.

CAYENNE PEPPER

Are you a hot salsa or chili fan? Then you'll want to learn more about the virtues of hot peppers. These ripe fruits of the *Capsicum* genus are widely used as a popular spice, but hot peppers are also dried and powdered or tinctured for medicinal purposes.

Cayenne stimulates digestion and muscle movement in the intestines, which helps restore deficient digestive secretions and aids absorption of food nutrients. (Stomach acid tends to decline with age, and some cases of poor digestion are related to this lack of acid.) Cayenne also stimulates circulation and blood flow to the peripheral areas of the body. Because of its ability to stimulate digestion and circulation, cayenne is often added to a wide variety of herbal remedies: It improves the absorption and circulation of the other herbs throughout the body.

Have you ever gone after the chips and salsa with gusto and then felt flushed and drippy in the nose? Cayenne warms the body and stimulates the release of mucus from the respiratory passages. Anyone who has eaten much cayenne knows hot peppers can clear the sinuses and cause sweating. Cayenne can actually raise the body temperature a bit as it stimulates circulation and blood flow to the skin. An herb, such as cayenne or ginger, that promotes fever and sweating has a diaphoretic action. This action can help "break a fever" and relieve colds and congestion. Fever is a natural and necessary phenomena generated by the body to fight bacteria and viruses. It is a misconception that fever is harmful or undesired; only very high or prolonged fevers are dangerous. Fevers speed up metabolic processes to increase production of disease-fighting white blood cells.

Cayenne has become a popular home treatment for mild high blood pressure and high blood cholesterol levels. Cayenne preparations prevent platelets from clumping together and accumulating in the blood, allowing the blood to flow more easily. Since it is thought to help improve circulation, it's often used by those who have slow metabolisms due to low thyroid function or those who are always cold or have cold hands and feet.

The source of cayenne's heat is capsaicin, the fiery phenolic resin found in most hot peppers. Capsaicin causes nerve endings to release a chemical known as substance P. Substance P transmits pain signals from the body back to the brain. When capsaicin causes substance P to flood out of the cells, we experience a sensation of warmth or even extreme heat. When the nerve endings have lost all of their substance P, no pain signals can be transmitted to the brain until the nerve endings accumulate more substance P. For this reason, topical cayenne pepper products are popular for the treatment of arthritis and bursitis and for temporary relief of pain from psoriasis, herpes zoster, and neuralgia (nerve pain). These cayenne preparations are most appropriate for longstanding chronic conditions, not acute inflammations.

Cayenne is often found in diet and weight-loss formulas. But can eating hot peppers really help you lose weight? Probably not, but cayenne may promote calorie burning, supporting your diet and exercise efforts. Because it aids in digestion and absorption of nutrients, cayenne can reduce appetite that is due to malabsorption, a common condition in overweight people.

To clear a head cold and relieve sinus pain and congestion, try drinking a cup of tea made with lemon and ginger or horseradish to which you've added a dash or two of cayenne pepper.

COMFORTING CHAMOMILE

Chamomile's medicinal secret is the volatile oil derived from its daisy-like flowers. An extract produced from the herb can reduce muscle spasms and inflammation of mucous membranes, making it a useful treatment for indigestion and menstrual cramps. Chamomile also contains chemicals that fight infections that cause minor illnesses.

Several studies indicate that chamomile is a good digestive aid. The herb contains a wide variety of active constituents. Bisabolol, one of its prime constituents, has anti-inflammatory properties and relaxes the smooth muscle lining of the digestive tract. In experimentally induced gastritis and other inflammations of the mucous membranes, chamomile consistently demonstrated quick and prolonged anti-inflammatory effects.

Chamomile may also help to prevent and heal ulcers. In one study, two groups of animals were fed a chemical known to cause ulcers. Animals that were also given chamomile developed significantly fewer ulcers than those who did not receive it. And animals that did develop ulcers recovered more quickly if they were fed chamomile.

As long ago as 1914, researchers were publishing papers proclaiming the herb's ability to block the actions of convulsants and other chemicals that cause spasms. Chamomile's sedating properties were documented in the 1950s.

For years, researchers attributed the herb's antispasmodic effect to the presence of flavonoids, such as apigenin and luteolin. But several recent trials have demonstrated that other constituents also contribute substantially to the herb's total sedative action. The importance of chamazulene and its precursor, matricin, has been demonstrated in nearly all of chamomile's actions.

The anti-inflammatory constituents of chamomile, including azulene, chamazulene, bisabolol, and matricin, appear to have distinct modes of action. Some of them are more powerful than others but perform for a shorter period of time; others are milder but perform for longer periods of time.

CINNAMON

You probably have some cinnamon powder or sticks somewhere in your kitchen. Cinnamon is a warming, stimulating, pleasant-tasting herb with many uses. Cinnamon is widely used as a flavoring agent for candy, toothpaste, mouthwashes, and bath and body products. In herbal teas, cinnamon improves the flavor of less palatable herbs. And, of course, it is a staple for baking and cooking.

Perhaps you use cinnamon more in the winter. Spiced cider, prepared by steeping cinnamon sticks and other herbs in apple cider, is a traditional winter beverage. Cinnamon has an affinity for the uterus and digestive organs because it improves circulation and energy flow in the abdomen. In Chinese medical philosophy, pain, cramps, and congestion are considered blocked energy. Cinnamon is thought to circulate *qi,* or vital energy, when it is stuck in the abdomen and move it to the rest of the body and to warm the body.

Cinnamon has a germicidal effect. Almost all highly aromatic herbs display some ability to kill germs and microbes. Cinnamon in mouthwashes and gargles can help kill germs and treat infections. You may use small amounts of cinnamon tea to relieve gas in the stomach. Larger amounts of cinnamon will stimulate and warm the stomach, promoting acidity and a laxative effect. Use of cinnamon as a laxative may prevent flatulence and intestinal cramping that can accompany use of some other laxatives.

FENNEL

This familiar culinary herb is considered a digestive aid and a carminative, or agent capable of diminishing gas in the intestines. It is recommended for numerous complaints related to excessive gas in the stomach and intestines, including indigestion, cramps, and bloating, as well as for colic in infants. Other Umbelliferae family members such as dill and caraway are also considered carminatives.

As an antispasmodic, fennel acts on the smooth muscle of the respiratory passages as well as the stomach and intestines, which is the reason that fennel preparations are used to relieve bronchial spasms. Since it relaxes bronchial passages, allowing them to open wider, it is sometimes included in asthma, bronchitis, and cough formulas.

Fennel is also known to have an estrogenic effect and has long been used to promote milk production in nursing mothers.

GINGER

This botanical and popular spice is native to southeast Asia but is readily available in the United States. Fresh ginger root is a staple in Asian cooking. Dried and powdered, it's used in medicine. Ginger is high in volatile oils, also known as essential oils. Volatile oils are the aromatic part of the plants that we so cherish. They are called volatile because as unstable molecules, they are given off freely into the atmosphere.

Ginger root powder may be useful in improving pain, stiffness, lack of mobility, and swelling. Larger dosages in the area of 3 or 4 grams of ginger powder daily appear most effective. But powder may not be the only effective form of ginger root—one study demonstrated benefits from the ingestion of lightly cooked ginger.

Ginger has also had a long history of use as a general remedy for forms of nausea like morning sickness, motion sickness, and nausea accompanying gastroenteritis (more commonly called stomach "flu"). As a stomach calming aid, ginger also reduces gas, bloating, and indigestion, and aids in the absorption and the body's use of other nutrients and medicines. It is also a valuable deterrent to intestinal worms, particularly roundworms. Ginger may even improve some cases of constant severe dizziness and vertigo. It may be both a therapy and a preventive treatment for some migraine headaches. Ginger also prevents platelets from clumping together in the bloodstream. This serves to thin the blood and reduce the risk of atherosclerosis and blood clots.

A warming herb, ginger can promote perspiration when ingested in large amounts. It stimulates circulation, particularly in the abdominal and pelvic regions, and can occasionally promote menstrual flow. If you are often cold, you can use warm ginger to help raise your body temperature.

ALLEVIATE ALLERGIES

Because honey contains trace amounts of pollen, some people believe consuming local honey derived from the pollen found in the flowers in your area (within a 10- to 15-mile radius of where you live) can help to alleviate allergy symptoms. Note: There's not enough pollen in the honey for you to experience a negative reaction—just enough to become better adjusted to it.

HONEY

Honey is the only food that includes all the nutrients necessary to sustain life. Honey and bee pollen contain water, as well as all 22 minerals and enzymes that the human body needs. Bonus: it's also fat- and cholesterol-free!

Honey is a fantastic option for many of life's minor maladies. For example:

- Honey can help wounds heal more rapidly. Apply it directly to a scratch, scrape, or small cut, and let it go to work.
- You may be able to fend off a migraine if you feel one coming on. Just take 1 teaspoon of honey as soon as you feel the warning signs. If it's already too late, take 2 teaspoons of honey with each meal until the headache subsides.
- Obtain relief from a hangover by taking 1 teaspoon of honey every hour until you feel better. The large quantity of fructose found in honey will help speed up the metabolism of alcohol in your system.

COLDS, COUGHS, AND SORE THROATS

- Help that sore throat—and promote the flow of mucus—by drinking a cup of hot tea mixed with 1 tablespoon of honey and 2 drops of lemon juice. This even works with plain hot water instead of tea! These are good tonics to help ease laryngitis, as well.
- More throat relief comes when honey soothes and vinegar kills bacteria. Whip up a batch of homemade cough syrup by mixing 1/4 cup each of apple cider vinegar and honey. Pour into a bottle or jar that can be sealed tightly. Take 1 tablespoon every 4 hours, shaking well before each dose.
- Sore throats respond well to this drink: In a glass of water, mix 1 teaspoon of honey, 3 tablespoons of lime juice, and 1 tablespoon of pineapple juice. Sip to obtain soothing relief.

SOOTHING A SICK STOMACH

Digest this suggestion: a teaspoon or two of honey mixed with milk can help improve digestion. The mixture works well either warm or cold, but some people swear by warm milk. You may also prevent indigestion by taking a spoonful of honey sprinkled with a bit of cinnamon before beginning a meal. Honey taken by itself or mixed with water, milk, or tea can remedy feelings of nausea too.

ADVICE FOR A LONG, HEALTHY LIFE

- What, me worry? The nutrients found in honey can help you feel calmer when you're experiencing anxiety or nervousness, so mix a spoonful of honey into your oatmeal, yogurt, or cereal to start your day off right. In fact, honey has incredible nutritional value, providing several antioxidants in addition to thiamin, niacin, riboflavin, pantothenic acid, and vitamin B6.

- Don't be down in the dumps! A straight shot of honey mixed into your favorite beverage is known to alleviate symptoms of depression.
- Fight fatigue with a mix of a teaspoon of honey in tepid water. The glucose in honey is quickly absorbed into your bloodstream and your brain, providing a quick pick-me-up.
- Honey has been known to boost athletic performance. Enjoy a tablespoon before your next workout.
- Take the edge off your appetite. Thirty minutes before each meal, drink a mixture of 2 teaspoons honey in a glass of water.
- Cool it down. Mix a teaspoon of honey and a teaspoon of vinegar in a glass of tepid water to treat heat exhaustion. This mixture of honey and vinegar is such a potent combination it can also be beneficial in lowering blood pressure, reducing the effects of eczema, and treating brittle fingernails and toenails.

HORSERADISH

Have you ever bitten into a roast beef sandwich and thought your nose was on fire? The sandwich probably contained horseradish. Even a tiny taste of this potent condiment seems to go straight to your nose. Whether on a sandwich or in a herbal preparation, horseradish clears sinuses, increases facial circulation, and promotes expulsion of mucus.

Horseradish is helpful for sinus infections because it encourages your body to get rid of mucus. One way a sinus infection starts is with the accumulation of thick mucus in the sinuses: Stagnant mucus is the perfect breeding ground for bacteria to multiply and cause a painful infection. Horseradish can help thin and move out older, thicker mucus accumulations. If you are prone to developing sinus infections, try taking horseradish the minute you feel a cold coming on. Herbalists also recommend horseradish for common colds, influenza, and lung congestion. Incidentally, don't view the increase of mucus production after horseradish therapy as a sign your cold is worsening. The free-flowing mucus is a positive sign that your body is ridding itself of wastes.

Horseradish has a mild natural antibiotic effect and it stimulates urine production. Thus, it has been used for urinary infections.

MARVELOUS MINT

Mint is one of the most reliable home remedies for an upset stomach. Grandmas have been handing out mints for centuries to treat indigestion, flatulence, and colic. The two types of mint you're most likely to encounter are spearmint and peppermint. Although they once were considered the same plant, peppermint actually is a natural hybrid of spearmint. It's also the more potent of the herbs.

Peppermint owes part of its healing power to an aromatic oil called menthol. Spearmint's primary active constituent is a similar but weaker chemical called carvone. Oil of peppermint contains up to 78 percent menthol. Menthol encourages bile (a fluid secreted by the liver) to flow into the duodenum, where it promotes digestion. Menthol also is a potent antispasmodic; in other words, it calms the action of muscles, particularly those of the digestive system.

Menthol's medicinal value has been borne out in numerous studies with animals and with humans. German and Russian studies show that peppermint not only helps to stimulate bile secretion but also may prevent stomach ulcers. The potent oil is also capable of killing myriad microorganisms that are associated with digestive and other problems. Recent studies, moreover, suggest that menthol may be useful in treating irritable bowel syndrome, a common but hard-to-treat digestive disorder in which the bowel contracts, causing a crampy type of adult colic.

MELONS

Melons come in a wide variety of shapes, sizes, and flavors, yet have certain healing nutrients in common. Their high levels of potassium benefit the heart. Some melons have health-boosting phytochemicals and top-notch amounts of vitamins C and A. Orange- fleshed melons, such as cantaloupe, are high in beta-carotene. One cup of melon cubes supplies nearly everyone's daily requirement for vitamin A. When studying endometrial cancer, researchers at the University of Alabama reported that women who did not have this cancer had eaten at least one food high in beta-carotene, such as cantaloupe, every day. The women who had endometrial cancer had eaten less than one beta-carotene food per week.

Watermelon's red pulp is teeming with a different carotenoid, lycopene. Lycopene is even more potent than beta-carotene at doing away with free radicals, those damaging molecules that can be the culprits in heart disease, cancer, and cataracts. High intakes of lycopene, though not watermelon itself as yet, are linked to a decreased incidence of prostate cancer.

NOTES ON NUTS

All nuts are healthful, but some are all-stars. Here are some highlights:

- **Walnuts** are one of the most-researched nuts, and all that study has concluded that they contain a unique combination of healthful fats and essential nutrients. Many scientists say this combination contributes to some remarkable benefits. Walnuts have more heart-healthful ALA omega-3 fatty acids than any other nut. A 2005 study done at the University of Texas Health Science Center showed that walnuts are a prime source of melatonin, an antioxidant that has been linked with a lower risk of cancer, less-severe heart disease, and improved brain function. Melatonin also has long been associated with better sleep.

- **Almonds** are amazing nuts that may help you slim down. A roundup of studies on almonds and weight shows that the body may not absorb the fat in almonds, so it doesn't contribute to weight gain. Almonds also have more of the antioxidant vitamin E than any other nut. You can satisfy 55 percent of your daily vitamin E needs in a one-and-a-half-ounce serving of almonds. And almonds contain alpha-tocopherol, the important type of vitamin E that the National Academy of Science deems the most active in the human body. Studies have linked alpha-tocopherol with lowered cholesterol levels, reduced risk of some cancers, fewer complications from diabetes, a Stronger immune system, and a healthier brain.

- **Peanuts**: According to a 2004 study published in the *American Journal of Clinical Nutrition,* women whose diet provided them with half of their fat (which was mostly unsaturated) coming from peanuts, peanut butter, and peanut oil reduced their risk of heart disease by 14 percent compared with women who ate a lower-fat diet that didn't include peanuts. The women who ate the diet that was rich in peanuts and unsaturated fat lost the same amount of weight as the women who ate the lower-fat diet. Peanuts are also a good source of fiber.

- **Pecans** are a potent source of antioxidants, zinc, copper, and magnesium. And one serving of pecans provides almost your entire daily requirement of manganese. Manganese aids in keeping your brain, blood, and bones healthy; helps your body better use calcium; and helps regulate blood-sugar levels. Manganese is considered an antioxidant, so it may help keep your arteries healthy and lower your risk of cancer.

NUTS AND CANCER

The abundant antioxidants in nuts might lower your risk of developing certain cancers. Antioxidants help protect cells from damage that can lead to cancer. Nuts contain several antioxidants, including vitamin E, ellagic acid, phytic acid, and selenium. Several studies have suggested that antioxidants might lower cancer risk. One of the largest was the Chinese Cancer Prevention Study, which was published in 1993. This trial tested a combination of beta-carotene, vitamin E, and selenium on men and women who were at high risk for developing stomach cancer. According to the results, this antioxidant combination not only substantially lowered the risk of stomach cancer, but it also lowered the overall risk of developing cancer.

Other studies have found that eating nuts lowers the risk of developing prostate cancer. The amount of scientific evidence collected has been enough for the American Institute of Cancer Research to suggest people at risk for prostate cancer include nuts in their diet. Similar studies on colon cancer in women have also found that eating nuts on a regular basis has protective benefits.

OATS

You might think oatmeal is the most boring bowl of breakfast food around, but oats are a fantastic source of healing nourishment. They contain starches, proteins, vitamins, and minerals, and though they contain some fat, they are low in saturated fat, which makes them a healthy choice. A serving of hot oat bran cereal provides about 4 grams of dietary fiber (health professionals recommend we consume 20 to 35 grams of fiber each day). Some types of dietary fiber bind to cholesterol, and since this form of fiber is not absorbed by the body, neither is the cholesterol. A number of clinical trials have found that regular consumption of oat bran reduces blood cholesterol levels in just one month. High fiber diets may also reduce the risk of colon and rectal cancer.

Oats have been used topically to heal wounds and various skin rashes and diseases. The familiar sticky-but-smooth consistency of cooked oats is emulated in many oat products; as a result they have mucilaginous, demulcent, and soothing qualities. Soaps and various bath and body products made from oats are readily available. Oatmeal baths are wonderful for soothing dry, flaky skin or allaying itching in cases of poison oak and chicken pox.

Because oats are believed to have a calming effect, herbalists recommend them to help ease the frustration and anxiety that often accompany nicotine and drug withdrawal. Oats contain the alkaloid gramine, which has been credited with mild sedative properties. Scientists have conducted clinical trials to determine whether oats may help treat drug addiction or reduce nicotine craving, but the evidence is inconclusive.

ONIONS

Although less research has been done on onions than on garlic, findings show the two have many of the same anticancer, cholesterol-lowering properties. A Harvard Medical School study showed that "good" HDL cholesterol climbed significantly when participants ate about half of a medium-sized raw onion each day. Cooked onion did not affect HDL levels.

Like garlic, onions also contain the smooth-muscle relaxant adenosine. This means that onions, too, may fight high blood pressure. They play a role in preventing blood clots as well, keeping blood platelets from sticking together and quickly dissolving clots that may have already formed. Researchers in India found that when raw or cooked onions were eaten along with fatty foods, the blood's clot-dissolving ability remained intact, which doesn't usually occur after fatty foods are eaten. It's a good idea, then, always to include onions when you eat that occasional high-fat meal. Be aware, though, that onions may cause heartburn to worsen in some people.

Onions have many substances that protect you from cancer. Scallions are particularly effective at fighting stomach cancer. Onions are also good at killing bacteria and viruses, which makes them useful for fending off colds and flu.

Studies suggest that the humble onion also helps insulin do its job by decreasing the liver's breakdown of insulin. This is good news for diabetics. Studies in India showed that onions—raw or cooked—help lower blood sugar levels.

PARSLEY

Parsley offers a cornucopia of disease-fighting vitamins and healing substances, especially when compared to the lettuces. More nutrient dense than most greens, parsley tops the chart in vitamins A and C and the minerals calcium and iron. Three ounces, or about ten sprigs, of parsley contain more folate than an orange, nearly a day's amount of vitamin C, and more vitamin A in the form of beta-carotene than an apricot. Parsley is a storehouse of minerals, too, with as much calcium as a serving of dark, leafy greens. It's also a good plant source of iron—it contains more iron than most. Parsley is packed full of potassium, too, which helps regulate heartbeat and blood pressure.

Parsley is brimming with strong antioxidants such as lutein, monoterpenes, and polyphenols, which help prevent cancerous cell changes. Polyphenols help stop cancerous nitrosamines from forming in the digestive tract.

Parsley is also known for its diuretic properties. Several of the substances in parsley and its seeds are used to treat bladder infections and kidney problems. Other compounds may reduce inflammation and increase circulation.

SAGE

"Why should anyone die who has sage in their garden?" This old saying speaks to the many conditions that can be treated with sage. The botanical name *Salvia* is from the Latin for "to save or to heal," as in the word "salvation."

People have been cooking with sage for thousands of years: Recipes for sage pancakes have been dated to the 5th century BC. Like most culinary herbs, sage is thought to be a digestive aid and appetite stimulant. You can use it to reduce gas in the intestines and, because it is also antispasmodic, to relieve abdominal cramps and bloating.

Sage contains phytosterols reported to have an estrogenic as well as a cooling action. Early and modern herbals list sage as a treatment for bright red, abundant uterine bleeding and for cramps that feel worse with heat applications and better with cold applications. You may also use sage to stop breast milk production when weaning a child from breast-feeding.

The drying effect that helps dry up milk and its reported cooling action also make sage useful for treating diarrhea, colds, and excessive perspiration. It may be of value for menopausal hot flashes accompanied by profuse perspiration. Sage can dry up phlegm, and you can gargle with the tea to treat coughs and tonsil or throat infections. Sage also has been recommended as a hair rinse for dandruff, oily hair, or infections of the scalp.

Sage is an antioxidant and an antimicrobial agent. The volatile oils in sage kill bacteria, making the herb useful for all types of bacterial infections.

Sage may also help to lower blood sugar in people with diabetes who consume it regularly.

SOY GOOD

When you think soy, you probably think tofu. But there's more to soy—and it's worth considering. The evidence linking soy protein and heart-disease prevention was so compelling that the Food and Drug Administration approved a health claim for use on food labels stating: "25 grams of soy protein per day, as part of a diet low in saturated fat and cholesterol, may reduce the risk of heart disease."

For many, getting this much soy in the diet is a challenge. Fortunately, soy foods are becoming more widely available and versatile, so the choices extend far beyond the traditional tofu and soy milk. For instance, a simple substitution of soy flour for up to 30 percent of all-purpose flour is an easy way to sneak in soy. Soy protein isolate, a powdered form of soy, can be added to a smoothie, sprinkled over cereal, or mixed in a casserole dish. Even easier and especially good for the soy wary are the veggie burgers, energy bars, breakfast cereals, and snack foods made from soy commonly available today.

SPINACH

Spinach's beautiful deep green color is a tip-off that it contains plenty of beta-carotene; those orange and red carotene pigments are hiding beneath the dark green chlorophyll. Spinach is also an excellent source of vitamin C, folate, and iron.

Spinach is a cornucopia of cancer fighters. For example, it has triple the amount of lutein and four times the amount of beta-carotene as broccoli. These antioxidants not only help prevent cancer, heart disease, and cataracts, but also boost the immune system. One study found that eating spinach more than twice a week was correlated with reduced risk of breast cancer. This vegetable contains a lot of folate, too. McGill University researchers found that folate improves serotonin levels in the brain, inducing a feeling of well-being. A daily dose of cooked spinach alleviated depression in study participants.

Spinach has the mineral manganese, too, which works with other minerals to strengthen bones. Although spinach is rich in calcium, the body is not able to absorb much of it. That's because spinach contains a compound called oxalic acid that binds with calcium, making it unavailable to the body. People who are prone to developing the most common type of kidney stones will want to limit their intake of spinach and rhubarb because the oxalic acid in these foods can promote the formation of stones.

SWEET POTATOES

Sweet potatoes are among the unsung heroes of healthy eating. Nutrient-packed with only a few calories, sweet potatoes support immune function, eyesight, heart health, and cancer protection.

Teeming with beta-carotene, sweet potatoes outrank carrots by far in this healthful nutrient. This beneficial antioxidant wages a continuous battle against free radicals and the diseases they trigger, including cancer. In a study at Harvard University, people who ate 3/4 cup cooked sweet potatoes, carrots, or spinach every day (all foods high in beta-carotene) had a 40 percent lower risk of experiencing a stroke. Researchers theorized that this nutrient protects blood cholesterol from undergoing damage from oxygen molecules. Damaged cholesterol begins the artery-clogging process. Other studies show that the more beta-carotene and vitamin A stroke patients have in their bloodstream, the less likely they are to die from the stroke and the more likely they are to make a full recovery.

All this beta-carotene also promotes healthy eyes and vision, since much of it gets turned into vitamin A as the body needs it. This wonder nutrient also works with certain white blood cells, tuning up your immune system to fight off colds, flu, and other illnesses.

Sweet potatoes rank right up with bananas as a source of potassium, the heart-friendly nutrient. These colorful roots are a surprisingly good source of vitamin C.

SWISS CHARD

This gently flavored vegetable is chock-full of beta-carotene and its relatives lutein and zeaxanthin, all potent disease fighters and immune boosters. The minerals potassium and magnesium, along with vitamin C, also hide in these beautifully colored, crinkled leaves.

Chard's carotenoids are strong protectors against cancer, heart disease, strokes, cataracts, and maybe even aging. Studies have not addressed whether eating chard confers these same protective benefits. Some researchers believe that antioxidants such as these prevent wear and tear on cells, thus reducing the number of times they need to reproduce within a person's lifetime and possibly slowing down the aging process. Chard also contains reasonable amounts of vitamin C, another antioxidant.

Even though chard is full of calcium and iron, like spinach, it's not very absorbable. Chard, too, is rich in oxalic acid, which binds these minerals.

Some people shy away from chard, having heard that it is high in sodium. One-half cup cooked chard does contain 158 mg of sodium, but this is just a fraction of the daily maximum recommended of 2400 mg. (However, our bodies only need 200 mg per day.) Processed foods such as crackers, chips, canned soups, and lunchmeats have many times more sodium than chard, and often without the plethora of healing nutrients.

TEA

Tea has long been considered a healthful drink, and even thousands of years ago it was prescribed for a wide variety of ailments. Now research is revealing the science behind the ancient wisdom. Tea has healing properties that can help prevent diseases as dissimilar as heart disease and cancer. Tea has three active ingredients that contribute to its healing power—flavonoids, fluoride, and caffeine. But the flavonoids are responsible for most of tea's health benefits.

GO GREEN WITH FLAVONOIDS

Research has shown an indisputable link between eating plant foods and good health. Vegetables and fruits contain an array of vitamins, minerals, and phytochemicals (plant compounds that have health-protective and disease-preventive properties). Tea, which comes from the *Camellia sinensis* plant, also has an abundance of phytochemicals.

There are thousands of phytochemicals in plants. Tea leaves contain a subgroup called polyphenols, or tea polyphenols, that include flavonoids. Polyphenols—including flavonoids—are powerful antioxidants, which are critical to your health because they act as a kind of defense system for your body. Antioxidants help neutralize destructive forms of oxygen or nitrogen known as free radicals, which are unstable molecules

TIME AND TEMPERATURE

One 2006 study in Taiwan found that the hotter the water, the faster the tea leaves would release antioxidants and caffeine into the brew. Steeping in cold water takes longer to produce a brew with the same level of antioxidants and caffeine.

101

that steal electrons from the molecules of healthy cells. Antioxidants protect cells by binding to free radicals and neutralizing them before they can damage DNA or other cell components. In addition to their antioxidant activity, flavonoids can also help regulate how cells function.

Tea is particularly high in flavonoids—higher than many vegetables or fruits. Tea provides about 83 percent of the total intake of flavonoids in the American adult diet, followed by citrus fruit juices (4 percent), and wine (2 percent), according to a 2007 study in the *American Journal of Nutrition*. Among the foods and beverages tested, black tea provides the largest number of flavonols—a type of flavonoid—in the U.S. diet (32 percent), according to scientists in the Nutrient Data Laboratory at the USDA Agricultural Research Service.

FLAVONOID LEVELS IN TEA — THE UPS AND DOWNS

There are thousands of flavonoids, but one type, called catechins, is currently in the limelight. Of special interest is epigallocatechin gallate (EGCG), a compound that is thought to be an especially powerful antioxidant. Researchers believe EGCG may be a key to the development of new drugs or complementary therapies to treat disease. Other important tea catechins include epicatechin (EC), epigallocatechin (EGC), and epicatechin gallate (ECG).

Green and white tea have an abundance of EGCG—more than black or oolong, both of which contain many other types of antioxidants that scientists have studied for their healing benefits. In fact, a cup of green tea has more catechins than an apple, according to the USDA Database for the Flavonoid Content of Selected Foods, 2007.

Different kinds of tea have different kinds of flavonoids. That's important because different flavonoids appear to play different roles in protecting the body from disease. While green tea has the most EGCG, black and oolong teas have more of the complex flavonoids called thearubigins and teaflavins. These are formed during the fermentation process and have been found to offer protection against heart attacks and cardiovascular disease.

Black, green, and oolong teas are a good source of the flavonols kaempferol, quercetin, and myricetin, which help relax blood vessels, improve blood flow, and reduce inflammation in cells, among other benefits.

CAFFEINE

Caffeine is a stimulant that increases heart rate, makes you alert, and revs up metabolism. All *Camellia sinensis* teas naturally contain caffeine, but the amount varies depending on the grade and type of tea, whether it is brewed from loose leaves or a tea bag, and how long it is brewed. Black tea has the most caffeine (42 to 72 mg per 8 ounces) while green, white, and oolong teas have less (9 to 50 mg per 8 ounces). Compare those amounts with the caffeine content of coffee, which has 110 to 140 mg per 8 ounces. Decaffeinated teas only have 1 to 4 mg per 8 ounces.

MINDING YOUR MONEY

In ancient China, green tea was thought to provide mental clarity, and now evidence of that is turning up in laboratory studies.

Experiments on mice and rat brain cells show that green tea antioxidants seem to prevent the formation of an Alzheimer's-related protein, beta-amyloid, which accumulates in the brain as plaque and leads to memory loss. This finding has been duplicated in a number of other cell-culture experiments. In one of these types of studies the antioxidants in black tea also were protective, although not as much as those in green tea.

In humans, green tea has been associated with a lower risk of dementia and memory loss. A Japanese study published in 2006 in the *American Journal of Clinical Nutrition* surveyed more than 1,000 people older than age 70. Those who drank two or more cups a day of green tea were half as likely to develop dementia and memory loss as those who drank fewer than two cups per week. This effect was much weaker for black and oolong teas.

THYME

Another secret weapon from the spice cabinet, thyme has a long and varied history of both medicinal and culinary use. With its strong antibacterial actions, it has found its way into numerous formulas for respiratory, digestive, skin, and other infections. Its antiseptic properties also make it suitable as a disinfectant cleanser and an atmospheric purifier. Before the days of refrigeration, a drop of thyme volatile oil was placed in a gallon of milk to keep it from spoiling. During the plague, townspeople gathered to burn large bundles of thyme and other herbs to keep the dreaded disease from their town. Early European physicians at one time carried aromatic thyme extracts with them as they visited the sick to prevent spreading disease or becoming ill themselves. Modern studies conducted in French hospitals show that simply introducing the aroma of thyme extracts into the air helps kill germs.

You can drink thyme tea for relief from coughs, bronchitis, and common colds. (Combining thyme with licorice or mint improves the flavor.) Thyme has a pronounced effect on the respiratory system; in addition to fighting infections, it dries mucous membranes and relaxes spasms of the bronchial passages. The ability of thyme to relax bronchial spasms makes it effective for coughs, bronchitis, emphysema, and asthma. Its drying effect makes it useful to reduce the abundant watering of the eyes and nose associated with hay fever and other allergies. And gargling with thyme tea can reduce swelling and pus formation in tonsillitis.

Thyme has been used to combat parasites such as hookworms and tapeworms within the digestive tract. It is also useful to treat yeast infections.

SAY YES TO YOGURT

Yogurt was a long-established staple in Eastern Europe and the Middle East before it reached our shores. And there was a time when yogurt eaters in this country were considered "health nuts." Our attitudes have changed considerably.

Yogurt may not be the miracle food some have claimed, but it certainly has a lot to offer in the health department. Besides being an excellent source of bone-building calcium, it is believed that the bacterial cultures, Lactobacillus bulgaricus and Streptococcus thermophilus, that are used to make yogurt carry their own health benefits. For example, research has suggested that eating yogurt regularly helps boost the body's immune system function, warding off colds and possibly even helping to fend off cancer. It is also thought the friendly bacteria found in many types of yogurt can help prevent and even remedy diarrhea.

For people who suffer from lactose intolerance, yogurt is often well tolerated because live yogurt cultures produce lactase, making the lactose sugar in the yogurt easier to digest. Be sure to check the label on the yogurt carton for the National Yogurt Association's Live and Active Cultures (LAC) seal. This seal identifies products that contain a significant amount of live and active cultures. But don't look to frozen yogurt as an option; most frozen yogurt contains little of the healthful bacteria.

HERBS AND SUPPLEMENTS

While many dismiss the use of herbs for healing, the use of botanicals is well rooted in medical practice. Ancient doctors methodically collected information about herbs and developed well-defined pharmacopoeias to treat a variety of ailments. More than a quarter of all drugs used today contain active ingredients derived from the same ancient plants. It's estimated that nearly 80 percent of the world's population use herbs for some aspect of primary healthcare. In the United States, more than 1,500 botanicals are sold as dietary supplements.

Like all medicines, botanicals may or may not offer positive health benefits, and some even may pose serious health threats. While the uncertain outcomes of modern medicine are generally accepted among health professionals, the same philosophy doesn't hold true for herbs.

ALFALFA

Herbalists often recommend alfalfa preparations as a potent nutritive in cases of malnutrition, debility, and prolonged illness. Alfalfa contains substances that bind to estrogen receptors in the body. Because alfalfa may provide some estrogenic activity when the body's hormone levels are low and compete for estrogen binding sites when hormone levels are high, alfalfa is said to be hormone balancing.

Both alfalfa sprouts and leaf preparations may help lower blood cholesterol levels. The saponins in alfalfa seem to bind to cholesterol and prevent its absorption. Blood cholesterol levels of animals fed alfalfa saponins for several weeks have been observed to decline. Alfalfa also has been studied for its ability to reduce atherosclerosis, or plaque buildup, on the insides of artery walls. Alfalfa is high in vitamins A, C, niacin, riboflavin, folic acid, and the minerals calcium, magnesium, iron, and potassium. Alfalfa also contains bioflavonoids.

BILBERRY

If you eat whortleberries and cream in England, you're getting a healthy dose of bilberries. Bilberries and huckleberries are popular food for hikers and forest birds and animals. The berries also make good dyes and very tasty jellies and jams. These berries freeze quite well, so you can harvest them in the summer and store them for year-round consumption.

Both the leaves and the ripe fruit of the bilberry and related berry species have long been a folk remedy for treating diabetes. Traditionally, people used the leaves to control blood sugar. While the leaves can lower blood sugar, they do so by impairing a normal process in the liver. For this reason, use of the leaves is not recommended for long-term treatment.

The berry, on the other hand, is recommended for people with diabetes. The berries do not lower blood sugar, but their constituents may help improve the strength and integrity of blood vessels and reduce damage to these vessels associated with diabetes and other diseases such as atherosclerosis (calcium and fat deposits in arteries). The berries contain flavonoids. The blue-purple pigments typical of this family are due to the flavonoid anthocyanin.

With their potent antioxidant activity, anthocyanins protect body tissues, particularly blood vessels, from oxidizing agents circulating in the blood. In the same way that pipes rust as a result of an attack by chemicals, various chemicals in our environment—pollutants, smoke, and chemicals in food—can bind to and oxidize blood vessels. Two common complications of diabetes, diabetic eye disease (retinopathy) and kidney disease (nephropathy), often begin when the tiny capillaries of these organs are injured by the presence of excessive sugar. Antioxidants allow these harmful oxidizing agents to bind to them instead of to body cells, preventing the agents.

Bilberry extracts may also reduce the tingling sensations in the extremities associated with diabetes. Several studies have shown that bilberry extracts stimulate blood vessels to release a substance that helps dilate (expand) veins and arteries. Bilberries help keep platelets from clumping together, which thins the blood, prevents clotting, and improves circulation.

Bilberry preparations seem particularly useful in treating eye conditions, so in addition to diabetic retinopathy, they are also used to treat cataracts, night blindness, and degeneration of the macula, the spot in the back of the eye that enables sharp focusing.

BLACK COHOSH

If you ache—whether from menstrual cramps, an injury, or a condition such as rheumatism—black cohosh may be the herb you need. Black cohosh acts as an antispasmodic to muscles, nerves, and blood vessels and as a muscle anti-inflammatory. It contains the anti-inflammatory salicylic acid (the base for the active ingredient in aspirin), among other constituents, and has been used for an assortment of muscular, pelvic, and rheumatic pains.

Black cohosh seems particularly effective for uterine cramps and muscle pain caused by nervous tension and pains accompanied by stiffness, soreness, and tight sensations of contraction. Native Americans used it for female and muscular conditions as well as fatigue, sore throat, arthritis, and rattlesnake bites. Early American physicians used black cohosh for female reproductive problems, including menstrual cramps and bleeding irregularities, as well as uterine and ovarian pain.

Black cohosh is used as an emmenagogue, an agent that promotes menstrual or uterine bleeding. Herbalists consider it a sedative emmenagogue, meaning it promotes blood flow when uterine tension, cramps, and congestion hinder flow. Black cohosh relaxes the uterus, especially when tension is caused by anxiety. Black cohosh is believed to act on the uterus by improving muscle tone, so it is useful for preventing miscarriage and premature labor. The herb is also recommended for women who have had difficult labors, and in those cases it is administered in small doses in the last trimester of pregnancy to prepare the uterus for delivery. It decreases labor pain by promoting more efficient contractions. When contractions during labor are weak, or for severe after-pains following labor, black cohosh is used.

The herb is also thought to have an estrogenic effect because its constituents bind to estrogen receptors in the body. The binding of a plant constituent to an estrogen receptor can increase estrogen activity in the affected tissues. This hormonal activity may improve uterine problems, such as poor uterine tone, menstrual cramps, and postmenopausal vaginal dryness. One recent study evaluated the effects of black cohosh and a placebo in 110 menopausal women. The women were given 8 milligrams of black cohosh or the placebo every day for eight weeks, and then blood levels of hormones were checked. The results showed that black cohosh has an estrogenic effect that could particularly benefit postmenopausal women.

Black cohosh is also a mild stomach tonic credited with alterative action. (An alterative is an agent capable of improving the absorption of nutrients and the elimination of wastes by the digestive tract.) Its sweet and bitter flavors stimulate digestion. Black cohosh has been shown to dilate peripheral blood vessels and sometimes improve elevated blood pressure. Early physicians also used black cohosh for serious infectious diseases, including whooping cough, scarlet fever, and smallpox. In China, the Chinese species, *Cimicifuga foetida,* is used for measles in addition to headache and gynecologic problems.

BLUE COHOSH

Blue cohosh is used primarily for uterine weakness and as a childbirth aid. It is considered a uterine stimulant in most circumstances because it improves uterine muscle tone. But blue cohosh also has an antispasmodic effect on cramps. Because of its dual actions, herbalists describe blue cohosh as a uterine tonic. The alkaloid methyl cytisine found in blue cohosh is thought to be antispasmodic, while the triterpenoid saponin hederagenin is thought to provide the increased uterine tone.

Blue cohosh is also classified as an emmenagogue, meaning it stimulates menstrual flow. It dilates blood vessels in the uterus and promotes circulation in the pelvis, making it helpful for women who experience scanty, spotty menstrual flow; irregular periods; and difficult, painful periods. Blue cohosh seems to work best for women who experience more painful menstrual cramps the first day of their period. You may use blue cohosh to relieve menstrual cramps and to treat a weak, worn-out, or sluggish-acting uterine muscle—indicated by no cramps or weak cramps, but prolonged bleeding; weak pelvic, abdominal, and thigh muscles; and an aching, dragging sensation during the menstrual period. Blue cohosh also may be useful in cases of breast tenderness and abdominal pain caused by fluid retention.

Blue cohosh helps correct uterine prolapse (sagging of the uterus in the pelvic cavity). This condition may stem from multiple childbirths or tissue laxity due to overweight or obesity. Blue cohosh also may help the uterus shrink back to its appropriate size after childbirth.

The herb has long been used by herbalists to prepare the uterus for childbirth. It is often combined with other botanicals (historically, black cohosh, motherwort, and partridge berry). The formula is taken in the last trimester of pregnancy to promote smooth, efficient labor and delivery, and rapid involution of the uterus (returning of the uterus to its normal size). While some sources state that blue cohosh is contraindicated during pregnancy, many herbalists and women have used blue cohosh safely and effectively during late pregnancy. This herb should not be used during early pregnancy, and it should be used during late pregnancy only under the supervision of a physician or skilled herbalist.

Blue cohosh is a diuretic—an agent that promotes urination—and a weak diaphoretic—an agent that raises body temperature and promotes sweating—which may help break a fever.

BURDOCK

Burdock is a perennial whose roots, and sometimes its seeds, are used widely in herbal medicine to support liver function and as a cleansing botanical. Like dandelion and yellow dock, burdock roots are bitter and thus capable of stimulating digestive secretions and aiding digestion. These roots are referred to as "alterative" agents—capable of enhancing digestion and the absorption of nutrients and supporting the elimination of wastes. Any botanical capable of these important actions can attain far-reaching improvements in a variety of complaints.

Burdock may also be useful in treating a variety of skin conditions, including acne and dryness, especially when these complaints are due to poor diet, constipation, or liver burden. The liver plays an important role in removing impurities from the blood, producing bile to digest fats, metabolizing hormones, and storing excess carbohydrates, in addition to its other functions. Everything absorbed from the digestive tract goes directly to the liver to be filtered, so when you eat foods that contain pesticides, preservatives, artificial coloring and the like, you give your liver extra work to do. A high-fat diet also forces your liver to work harder because it must break down the fat with the bile it produces. Add to this all of the potential toxins we are exposed to in daily life that the liver must remove from the bloodstream (car exhaust, nicotine, prescription drugs, alcohol, cleaning products, industrial toxins, etc.), and you can see how the liver can become overworked or burdened.

Burdock is useful in cases of hormone imbalance that are not attributable to uterine fibroids, cancer, or other diseases. Many conditions such as premenstrual syndrome, fibroids, and endometriosis are associated with excess estrogen levels. Because of its alterative action, and because of the small amount of plant steroids it contains, burdock can help improve the liver's ability to metabolize hormones such as estrogen and thereby improve symptoms associated with hormonal imbalance.

Burdock contains a starch-like substance called inulin that is easily digested. Inulin is also found in other Compositae family members—dandelion, elecampane, and Jerusalem artichokes. Burdock has been recommended to people with diabetes because studies show inulin is easier for them to metabolize than other starches. Inulin breaks down into the simple sugar fructose, which does not require insulin to move into cells.

CRAMP BARK

As its name implies, cramp bark is useful to ease uterine cramps. But as a muscle relaxant, it also affects other organs, including the intestines and the skeletal muscles. Cramp bark is considered the most potent uterine antispasmodic of the various Viburnum species because it contains more of the antispasmodic constituent scopoletin. Cramp bark also contains more antispasmodic volatile oils than other species. Cramp bark usually works rapidly for simple menstrual cramps. If it fails to relieve symptoms, the discomfort is probably not due to uterine muscle spasm but to inflammation or irritation of the uterus or ovaries, endometrial infection, or cysts. Cramp bark's close relative, black haw, is also useful for uterine cramps, congestion, irritation in the uterus, and ovaries with radiating pains and may be better indicated for those types of complaints.

Cramp bark has been used to halt contractions during premature labor. It has also been used in the last trimester of pregnancy to build up uterine muscles and ensure an easy labor. Be sure to consult with an experienced herbalist or naturopathic physician before taking any botanicals during pregnancy.

The antispasmodic constituents in cramp bark also may lower blood pressure by relaxing vessel walls. When taken in large dosages (30 drops or more every two or three hours), cramp bark may reduce leg cramps, muscle spasms, or pain from a stiff neck.

DANDELION

Gathered early, after the spring's first warm spell, the leaves and roots are used as a spring tonic and to stimulate digestion and vitality after a long winter. Dandelion greens have also been used as a diuretic, an agent that promotes the loss of water from the body through urination. Their diuretic effect can make dandelion greens helpful in lowering blood pressure and relieving premenstrual fluid retention.

Dandelion roots contain inulin and levulin, starch-like substances that may help balance blood sugar, as well as a bitter substance (taraxacin) that stimulates digestion. The very presence of a bitter taste in the mouth promotes the flow of bile from the liver and gallbladder, and hydrochloric acid from the stomach. Bitters have been used for centuries in many countries before meals as a digestive stimulant. Do you avoid bitter-tasting foods? Many people do, but this may not reflect a balanced appetite. According to Asian philosophies, the diet should contain foods that are sweet, salty, sour, and bitter. The few bitter tastes Westerners embrace are coffee, wine, and beer, which may have something to do with the higher incidence of digestive diseases in Western cultures compared with Asian cultures.

Dandelion leaves are also rich in minerals and vitamins, particularly calcium and vitamins A, C, K, and B2 (riboflavin). Besides the stimulating bitter substances, dandelion roots also contain choline, another liver stimulant. Dandelion roots make wonderful colon cleansing and detoxifying medications because any time digestion is improved, the absorption of nutrients and the removal of wastes from the body improves as well. Many people could use a little extra support for the liver: We are inundated daily with chemicals and substances that the liver must process. The liver must filter impurities from the bloodstream—all the car exhaust, paints, cleaners, solvents, preservatives, pesticide residues, drugs, alcohol, and other toxins we encounter can begin to tax the liver. Add a diet high in fat, which the liver must emulsify with bile, and a person could experience physical symptoms from this burden on the liver. Rough dry skin and acne, constipation, gas and bloating, frequent headaches, and premenstrual syndrome are all potential symptoms of an overburdened liver.

ECHINACEA

This showy perennial was used by the Native Americans and adopted by the early settlers as a medicine. Members of the medical profession in early America relied heavily on echinacea, but it fell from favor with the advent of pharmaceutical medicine and antibiotics. Many physicians are rediscovering the benefits of echinacea today. Many forms of echinacea are available to choose from; Germany has registered more than 40 different echinacea products.

Long used for infectious diseases and poor immune function, echinacea extractions are also used today to help treat cancer, chronic fatigue syndrome, and AIDS. Research has shown echinacea stimulates the body's natural immune function. It also increases both the number and the activity of white blood cells, raises the level of interferon, and stimulates blood cells to engulf invading microbes. Echinacea also increases the production of substances the body produces naturally to fight cancers and disease.

FEVERFEW

Feverfew is used to relieve headaches, particularly vascular headaches such as migraines. Doctors aren't sure what causes migraines, but they know these severe headaches involve blood vessel changes. One theory suggests that migraines occur when the blood vessels in the head expand and press on the nerves, causing pain. Another theory proposes that these headaches occur as the blood vessels react to outside stimuli by affecting blood flow to various parts of the brain. Feverfew relaxes tension in the blood vessels in the brain and inhibits the secretion of substances that cause pain or inflammation (such as histamine and serotonin). Studies confirm feverfew's effectiveness as a migraine remedy.

Although some herbalists believe feverfew is most effective when used long-term to prevent chronic migraines, some people find it helpful when taken at the onset of a headache. Besides vascular headaches, feverfew may also benefit those who experience premenstrual headaches, which are often due to fluid retention and hormonal effects.

Feverfew is also reported to reduce fever and inflammation in joints and tissues. Some physicians recommend it to relieve menstrual cramps and to facilitate delivery of the placenta following childbirth.

Feverfew contains the substance parthenolide, which has been credited with inhibiting the release of serotonin, histamine, and other inflammatory substances that make blood vessels spasm and become inflamed. Reportedly, the amount of parthenolide varies from plant to plant, so it is wise to know how much of this active ingredient a feverfew product contains before you buy it. One study of commercially available feverfew products found that most of them contained no parthenolide at all: They were dried herbs, and because parthenolide is volatile, it had all evaporated. Look for a product that contains 0.2 percent parthenolide.

GINKGO

Gingko leaf has been the subject of extensive modern clinical research in Europe. Its most striking clinical effect is its ability to dilate blood vessels and improve circulation and vascular integrity in the head, heart, and extremities. Reduced circulation to the head is responsible for many of the mental and neurologic symptoms of aging, including memory loss, depression, and impaired hearing. Double-blind clinical trials—considered the most reliable method of scientific research—have shown that ginkgo can help ease these conditions when they are due to impaired circulation.

Ginkgo also has other actions on the brain, including strengthening the vessels and promoting the action of neurotransmitters—chemical compounds responsible for the transmission of nerve impulses between brain and other nerve cells.

Because it increases circulation in the heart and limbs, ginkgo may be useful for ischemic heart disease or intermittent claudication, conditions that can occur when blood flow to the muscles is reduced because atherosclerosis has narrowed the arteries. Ginkgo dilates the clogged arteries and allows more blood flow to the muscles. Ginkgo also thins the blood, reducing its tendency to clot, another benefit in atherosclerotic disease.

Constituents in ginkgo are also potent antioxidants with anti-inflammatory effects. A common current scientific theory attributes many of the signs of aging and chronic disease to the oxidation of cell membranes by radicals. These may arise from pollutants in the atmosphere or from the normal production of metabolic by-products and wastes. Antioxidant vitamins and other substances, including gingko, are currently being investigated for their ability to counter inflammation and destruction or damage to cells from oxidation.

AMERICAN AND ASIAN GINSENG

The enthusiasm over ginseng began thousands of years ago in China, where the Asian species of ginseng, Panax ginseng, grows. So valued was China's native species, the plant was overharvested from the wild, causing scarcity and increased demand. A mature woods-grown root of Panax ginseng will sometimes fetch $1,000 or more. A mature wild woods-grown root of Panax ginseng will sometimes fetch $200,000 or more!

When a similar species, Panax quinquefolius, was noted in the early American colonies, tons of the plant were immediately dug and exported to China. Many American pioneers made their living digging ginseng roots from moist woodlands. As a result, ginseng has become rare in its natural habitat in the United States as well. Ginseng is now cultivated in forests or under vast shading tarps.

Many people believe the cultivated ginseng has slightly different properties than the natural wild specimens. The Asian species is said to be the superior medicine compared with the American species, but the two species have slightly different applications. The Asian Panax ginseng is said to be a yang tonic, or more warming, while the American Panax quinquefolius is said to be a yin tonic, or more cooling. Both the ginseng and the quinquefolius species are qi tonics, or agents capable of strengthening qi, our vital life force.

Traditional Chinese medicine is very sophisticated, and its botanical therapies are fine-tuned accordingly. Panax ginseng, for example, might be recommended to warm and stimulate someone who is weak and cold from nervous exhaustion. Panax quinquefolius, on the other hand, is best for someone who is hot, stimulated, and restless from nervous exhaustion and feverish wasting disease. It is good for someone experiencing a lot of stress (and subsequent insomnia). American ginseng is used in China to help people recuperate from fever and the feeling of fatigue associated with summer heat.

GOLDENSEAL

The strong market demand for goldenseal is due to its reputed antimicrobial and mild anti-inflammatory properties. Its astringent properties also make it useful for treating conditions of the throat, stomach, and vagina when these tissues are inflamed, swollen, or infected. The yellow-pigmented powder also makes a good antiseptic skin wash for wounds and for internal skin surfaces, such as in the vagina and ear canal. Goldenseal eye washes have been used for simple conjunctivitis.

An anti-inflammatory and antimicrobial astringent, goldenseal is particularly effective on the digestive system—from the oral mucosa to the intestinal tract. It is helpful for canker sores in the mouth and as a mouth rinse for infected gums. For sore throats, goldenseal works well combined with echinacea and myrrh. Gargling with goldenseal is effective, too; extended surface contact with the infected area is ideal treatment. Irritable bowel diseases also benefit from the use of goldenseal when there is diarrhea and excessive intestinal activity and secretions. For general debility of the stomach and digestion, such a chronic gas, indigestion, and difficulty with absorption of nutrients, herbalists recommend a combination of equal parts goldenseal and cayenne pepper in tincture or capsules before meals on a regular basis. Goldenseal has been found useful in treating the many types of diarrhea commonly seen in AIDS patients. Weakened immune function makes people susceptible to intestinal and other infections; goldenseal can help prevent and treat these infections.

Goldenseal has been found to be effective against a number of disease-causing organisms, including Staphylococcus, Streptococcus, and Chlamydia species and many others. Berberine and related alkaloids in goldenseal have been credited with its antimicrobial effects. Berberine may be responsible for the increased white blood cell activity associated with goldenseal use, as well as its promotion of blood flow in the liver and spleen. Promoting circulation in these organs enhances their general function.

Berberine has been used recently in China to combat the depression of the white blood cell count that commonly follows chemotherapy and radiation therapy for cancer. Both human and animal studies suggest berberine may have potential in the treatment of brain tumors and skin cancers. Since goldenseal acts as an astringent to mucosal tissues, it has been recommended to treat oral cancers as well as abnormal cells in the cervix (cervical dysplasia) and cervical cancer. Goldenseal's astringent and immune-stimulating action seems to heal inflamed cells and eliminate abnormal cells. Goldenseal has the curious reputation as an herb people take before undergoing a drug test to ensure they pass. There is no logical basis for this; herbalist author and photographer Steven Foster cleared up this rumor when he pointed out it stemmed from the plot of a fictional murder mystery written by a prominent herbalist, John Uri Lloyd, almost a century ago.

HAWTHORN

Hawthorn is an important botanical cardiotonic (capable of producing and restoring the normal tone of the heart), and medications are made from the flowers and, especially, berries of the hawthorn tree. Hawthorn's many chemical constituents include the flavonoids—anthocyanidins and proanthocyanidins—which reduce blood vessel sensitivity to and damage from oxidizing agents. Various chemicals in our environment—pollutants, smoke, and chemicals in food—can bind to and damage the lining of blood vessels. Hawthorn improves the integrity of veins and arteries, enhancing circulation and nutrition to the heart, thus improving the function of the heart muscle itself. This action makes it useful for cases of angina (chest pain), atherosclerosis (a buildup of fat on the inside of artery walls), weakness and enlargement of the heart, high and low blood pressure, and elevated cholesterol levels. Hawthorn may also help control arrhythmias and palpitations. Early American Eclectic physicians suggested that hawthorn be used for valvular problems of the heart, especially when accompanied by a fast heart rate and nervousness. Modern herbalists continue to use hawthorn for such complaints.

HOPS

Hops are best known for their use as a bitter agent in brewing beer. But hops are also a nerve sedative and hormonal agent. Because they promote stomach secretions, bitter herbs are good digestive tonics. The bitter principles in hops are particularly useful for indigestion aggravated by stress or insufficient stomach acid and for gassiness and burping. Research has shown that hops may also help the body metabolize natural toxins such as those produced by bacteria.

Hops contain plant estrogens, and women who harvest hops flowers for an extended time sometimes develop menstrual-cycle abnormalities. Its estrogenic constituents make this plant useful to treat menopausal complaints, such as insomnia and hot flashes. You may also use hops for anxiety and nervous complaints or for indigestion and cramps resulting from anxiety. Use the tincture or tea before bed if you experience insomnia.

HORSETAIL

Horsetail is used medicinally to treat bladder infections and bladder weakness. Adults who experience occasional nocturnal incontinence (bed-wetting) may benefit from using horsetail preparations. The herb relieves a persistent urge to urinate.

Horsetail is classified as a diuretic, but sources differ as to its strength in this regard. Horsetail tea or tincture may help people who experience edema (fluid buildup) in the legs caused by such conditions as rheumatoid arthritis and circulatory problems. Because it contains silica and minerals, horsetail often is used to strengthen bone, hair, and fingernails—parts of the body that require high mineral levels. You may drink horsetail tea every day—for no longer than a month—if you've broken a bone. Horsetail also may be used by those who have wounds that do not heal well.

JUNIPER

With their warming, stimulating, and disinfecting actions, juniper berries have many medicinal uses. Juniper berries have an antiseptic effect and are often used in cases of chronic and repeated urinary tract infection. They are used in between flare-ups in those with frequent infections but not for acute cases of bladder infection.

Juniper stimulates urinary passages, causing the kidneys to move fluids faster. This is helpful if your kidneys are working sluggishly (such as with renal insufficiency), and urine is not flowing freely. But such stimulation would be disastrous if you had a raging kidney infection. Because of the myriad dangers, juniper must be used judiciously, starting with small, cautious dosages, and only under the supervision of an experienced practitioner. It also may be used for prolapse and weakness of the bladder or urethra.

Because juniper is indicated for chronic conditions associated with debility and lack of tone in the tissues, it is most often used for treating older people or those with chronic diseases. Both the aging process and prolonged disease are associated with loss of tone in tissues and organs. Since juniper is stimulating, it is useful in these situations.

Juniper berries also are recommended for joint pain, gout, rheumatoid arthritis, and nerve, muscle, and tendon disorders. The plant is used internally and topically for such complaints in small doses over several weeks. Take juniper for a week; then abstain for two.

Juniper's volatile oils have been concentrated and used topically for coughs and lung congestion. Its tars and resins have been isolated and used topically to treat psoriasis and other stubborn skin conditions. This treatment may irritate the skin, so you should dilute it and gradually increase the concentration. In both topical therapies, juniper has a warming, stimulating, and irritating action. Juniper also is considered to be a uterine stimulant, occasionally used by herbalists to improve uterine tone and late or slow-starting menstrual periods. Juniper is valuable for respiratory infections and congestion because the volatile oil in its berries opens bronchial passages and helps to expel mucus. Juniper's volatile oils also relieve gas in the digestive system and increase stomach acid when insufficient. Hydrochloric acid in the stomach is required to digest food, and insufficient acid leads to incomplete digestion, gassiness, and bloating.

LAVENDER

Lavender has been cherished for centuries for its sweet, relaxing perfume. Its name comes from the Latin root *lavare* meaning *to wash*, since lavender was frequently used in soaps and hair rinses.

Besides its importance as a fragrance, lavender is considered calming to nervous tension. Lavender oil is sometimes rubbed into the temples for head pain, added to bathwater for an anxiety-reducing bath, or put on a cotton ball and placed inside a pillowcase to treat insomnia. Lavender flowers are added to tea formulas for a pleasing, soothing aroma; the tea is sipped throughout the day to ease nervous tension. Lavender has a mildly sedating action and is also a weak antispasmodic for muscular tension.

Lavender may also alleviate gas and bloating in intestines as most herbs high in volatile oils are reported to do. One of lavender's volatile oils, linalool, has been found to relax the bronchial passages, reducing inflammatory and allergic reactions. Lavender is sometimes included in asthma, cough, and other respiratory formulas. Linalool is also credited as an expectorant and antiseptic.

Lavender is commonly added to soaps, perfumes, powders, and potpourri blends. Enormous quantities of lavender are steam-distilled to prepare the concentrated volatile oils, which are used in the perfume and cosmetic industry and are available in the pure form in health food stores and perfume shops. The volatile oils may be used topically and in the practice of aromatherapy (using essential oils to elicit a medicinal effect).

You can add dried lavender flowers to tea formulas. Briefly steep 1 teaspoon to 1 tablespoon flowers per cup of hot water. When infusing lavender, use a lid to prevent the volatile oils from escaping into the air.

LEMON BALM

Lemon balm is classified as a stimulating nervine, or nerve tonic, and though it has a soothing effect on the nervous system and alleviates anxiety, it is not a simple sedative. Lemon balm is particularly indicated for nervous problems that have arisen from longstanding stress and for anxiety accompanied by headache, sluggishness, confusion, depression, and exhaustion. Researchers have found that a mixture of lemon balm and valerian is as effective as some tranquilizers, without the side effects.

Lemon balm is also credited with an antiviral effect, and it seems particularly effective against the herpes virus. Lemon balm alleviates stomach gas and cramps and has a general antispasmodic effect on the stomach and intestines. It also relaxes the blood vessels, which helps to reduce blood pressure.

LICORICE

Licorice is used to treat a truly vast array of illnesses. In China especially, licorice is considered a superior balancing or harmonizing agent and is added to numerous herbal formulas. It is used to soothe coughs and congestion, reduce inflammation, soothe and heal ulcers and stomach inflammation, control blood sugar, and balance hormones. Licorice is great for healing canker sores and cold sores (herpes simplex virus type I). Licorice is a potent antiviral agent and can be used to treat flu, herpes, and other viruses. Licorice is also a strong anti-inflammatory agent and can be used to improve the flavor of other herbs. With all of these uses, it is no wonder that licorice finds its way into so many healing therapies.

Several modern studies have demonstrated the ulcer-healing abilities of licorice. Unlike most popular ulcer medications, such as cimetidine, licorice does not dramatically reduce stomach acid; rather, it reduces the ability of stomach acid to damage stomach lining by encouraging digestive mucosal tissues to protect themselves from acid. Licorice enhances mucosal protection by increasing mucous-secreting cells, boosting the life of surface intestinal cells, and increasing microcirculation within the gastrointestinal tract. This improves the health of the stomach lining and reduces damage from stomach acid. One study in Ireland showed a licorice extract to be a better symptom reliever than Tagamet for a number of ulcer patients.

The remarkably sweet saponin glycoside glycyrrhizin is what gives licorice its characteristic flavor. (Glycyrrhizin is 60 times sweeter than sugar.) Glycyrrhizin is also an anti-inflammatory, and licorice also has been used to treat inflammations of the lungs, bowels, and skin. Glycyrrhizin is one of the constituents found to prolong the length of time that cortisol, one of the adrenal hormones, circulates throughout the body. Among other actions, cortisol reduces inflammation. Anything that prolongs the life of cortisol naturally helps to reduce inflammation.

Many anti-inflammatory drugs are synthetic versions of cortisol. They control conditions such as asthma, arthritis, bowel disease, and eczema by suppressing the immune systems, which halts the body's ability to mount an inflammatory response. Licorice is not thought to suppress the immune system the way pharmaceutical steroids do. However, both pharmaceutical cortisones and licorice may cause the same side effects: weight gain, fluid retention, and as a possible result, high blood pressure. Still, if you use cortisone, prednisone, or a similar steroid, you should seek the advice of a naturopathic or other knowledgeable physician to determine whether your condition may be managed another way.

MARSHMALLOW

Mallow is used as a soothing demulcent to help heal skin, wounds, and internal tissues. The bladder responds particularly well to mallow preparations. With the help of a skilled herbalist, many people may improve chronic bladder infections and avoid repeated antibiotic therapy. Mallow also may be used for stomach irritation and ulcers, sore throats, coughs, and bronchitis. Mallow preparations may be used topically to treat abrasions, rashes, and inflammations.

MILK THISTLE

Milk thistle is a potent antioxidant: Research has found that it significantly increases levels of glutathione, which the liver uses to detoxify and metabolize harmful substances. In fact, milk thistle is used primarily to treat liver disorders, including cirrhosis and those caused by exposure to liver-damaging substances (such as alcohol and other drugs). The flavonoids in milk thistle appear to repair damaged liver cells, protect existing cells, and stimulate production of new liver cells. From a nasty hangover to a case of hepatitis, milk thistle helps the liver.

Milk thistle extracts have a preventive and therapeutic effect when taken orally and work particularly well when injected intravenously. The benefits of milk thistle extracts are demonstrated by improved symptoms in those with alcoholic liver disease and hepatitis and by improved liver function tests.

MOTHERWORT

Motherwort has been used for centuries to treat conditions related to childbirth. Motherwort has the ability to act as a galactagogue, meaning it promotes a mother's milk flow. It has also been used as a uterine tonic before and after childbirth. The herb contains a chemical called leonurine, which encourages uterine contractions. Motherwort is also claimed to be an emmenagogue, or an agent that promotes menstrual flow. It has been used for centuries to regulate the menstrual cycle and to treat menopausal and menstrual complaints.

Motherwort is also a mild relaxing agent and is often used by herbalists to treat such menopausal complaints as nervousness, insomnia, heart palpitations, and rapid heart rate. The herb may help heart conditions aggravated by nervousness. In such cases, motherwort combines well with blue cohosh and ginger tinctures.

Motherwort has sometimes been referred to as a cardiotonic. Motherwort injections were recently shown to prevent the formation of blood clots, which, of course, improves blood flow and reduces the risk of heart attack, stroke, and other diseases. It is good for hypertension because it relaxes blood vessels and calms nerves. Motherwort may also correct heart palpitations that sometimes accompany thyroid disease and hypoglycemia (low blood sugar). Motherwort is also useful for headache, insomnia, and vertigo. It is sometimes used to relieve asthma, bronchitis, and other lung problems, usually mixed with mullein and other lung herbs.

MYRRH

Myrrh stimulates circulation to mucosal tissues, especially in the bronchial tract, throat, tonsils, and gums. It is useful for bleeding gums, gingivitis, tonsillitis, sore throat (including strep throat), and bronchitis. The increased blood supply helps fight infection and speed healing when you have a cold, congestion, or infection of the throat or mouth. Myrrh is also valued as an expectorant, which means it promotes the expulsion of mucus in cases of bronchitis and lung congestion. Myrrh is best for chronic conditions with pale and swollen tissues rather than for acute, inflamed, red and dry tissues because it contains tannins, which have an astringent effect on tissues.

Myrrh may also promote menstrual flow and is recommended when menstruation is accompanied by a heavy sensation in the pelvis. In China, myrrh is considered a "blood mover." It may alleviate menstrual cramps.

NETTLES

Throughout early Europe, nettles were credited with nourishing and immune-stimulating properties. Nettle tea was used for intestinal weakness, diarrhea, and malnutrition—uses that persist to the present time. Nettles also act as a diuretic and are useful to treat kidney weakness and bladder infections. As a diuretic, nettles can help rid the body of excess fluid (edema) in persons with weakened hearts and poor circulation.

Nettles have also been used topically to treat eczema and skin rashes and soothe arthritic and rheumatic joints. In fact, the plant has been most widely studied for its value in the treatment of arthritis and gout. When uric acid, a product of protein digestion, accumulates in the joints and tissues, a very painful inflammatory condition known as gout can result. One tablespoon of fresh nettle juice several times a day has been shown to help clear uric acid from the tissues and enhance its elimination from the body.

Fresh nettle preparations sting a bit, and it is this sting that seems to have a healing effect: The reddening and stinging of the skin appear to reduce the inflammatory processes of both dermatologic (such as eczema) and rheumatic conditions (such as arthritis and gout). The tiny, stinging hairs contain formic acid and a bit of histamine. (Mosquitoes and biting ants also secrete formic acid, which is responsible for the familiar stinging and itching of their bites.) Nettles are also high in anti-inflammatory flavonoids, and they contain small amounts of plant sterols. They are extremely rich in vital nutrients, including vitamin D, which is rare in plants; vitamins C and A, and minerals, including iron, calcium, phosphorus, and magnesium.

Since nettles contain numerous nourishing substances, they are used in cases of malnutrition, anemia, and rickets and as a tonic to help repair wounds and broken bones. You can cook nettles and eat them as you would steamed spinach, for their taste and appearance are similar. Nettles are a healthy and tasty addition to scrambled eggs, pasta dishes, casseroles, and soups. You can also juice nettles and combine the juice with other fresh juices, such as carrot or apple juice, for weak, debilitated persons, such as cancer and AIDS patients. Nettle preparations have also been shown to be effective in controlling hay fever symptoms.

OREGON GRAPE

Berberis preparations are used extensively in herbal medicine for infections and to improve digestion and liver function: Oregon grape improves the flow of blood to the liver and acts as a bitter tonic, stimulating the flow of bile and intestinal secretions. For these reasons, Oregon grape is often used to treat jaundice, hepatitis, poor intestinal tone and function, and general gastrointestinal dysfunction. The berberine alkaloid has been shown to be of benefit for some patients with cirrhosis of the liver.

Oregon grape is also useful to treat colds, flu, and numerous infections. In the lab, it has been shown to kill or suppress the growth of some of the nastiest pathogens (disease-causing microbes): Candida and other fungi, Staphylococcus, Streptococcus, E. coli, Entamoeba histolytica, Trichomonas vaginalis, Giardia lamblia, Vibrio cholerae, and numerous others. Herbalists recommend it as an eyewash (since it must be highly diluted, don't try to make the eye preparations yourself), as a vaginal douche, or topically as a skin wash. The tincture is used to treat eczema, acne, herpes, and psoriasis. Oregon grape is an effective alternative to antibiotics in many situations. Check with your naturopathic physician or herbalist regarding the treatment of infectious conditions.

PASSION FLOWER

Passion flower has been used for anxiety, insomnia, restlessness, epilepsy, and other conditions of hyperactivity, as well as high blood pressure. Passion flower is also included in many pain formulas when discomfort is caused by muscle tension and emotional turmoil. In Europe the flowers are added to numerous pharmaceuticals to treat nerve disorders, heart palpitations, anxiety, and high blood pressure. Unlike most sedative drugs, passion flower has been shown to be non-addictive, although it is not a strong pain reliever.

PEPPERMINT

Peppermint is widely used as a food, flavoring, and disinfectant. As a medicine, peppermint is most well known for its effects on the stomach and intestines. Perhaps you've tried the various "tummy teas" available for stomach upset. Peppermint is a tasty way to relieve gas, nausea, and stomach pain due to an irritable bowel, intestinal cramps, or indigestion. Peppermint is a carminative—an agent that dispels gas and bloating in the digestive system—and an antispasmodic capable of relieving stomach and intestinal cramps. Peppermint can be used for too much stomach acid (hyperacidity) and gastroenteritis (nausea and stomach upset that we sometimes call stomach flu), and it is safe for infants with colic. When treating a baby with tummy cramps, you can give a teaspoon of peppermint tea if the baby will take it, or put a cloth soaked in warm peppermint tea on the infant's belly.

Peppermint is also used topically for the cooling and relaxing effect it has on the skin. Various muscle rubs and "ices" contain peppermint oil to reduce pain, burning, and inflammation. Like other volatile oils, peppermint oil is absorbed fairly well and can have a temporary pain-relieving effect on muscles and organs that are cramped and in spasm.

As with all essential oils, dilute this oil before putting it directly on your skin. Peppermint also allays itching temporarily. Rub a drop of diluted peppermint oil onto insect bites, eczema, and other itching lesions. Peppermint can help relieve some headaches, and you can rub peppermint oil onto the temples or scalp for a comforting therapy.

Menthol, the essential oil in peppermint, is credited with the herb's analgesic, antiseptic, antispasmodic, decongestant, and cooling effects. Menthol also helps subdue many disease-producing bacteria, fungi, and viruses, but because stronger herbal antimicrobials are available, peppermint is not usually the first choice of herbalists to treat serious infections. Peppermint tea can be used as a mouthwash for babies with thrush (yeast in the mouth) or for pregnant women who wish to avoid stronger herbs and medications.

RED CLOVER

Have you ever taken a nip of nectar from the tiny florets of this familiar meadowland plant? The bees certainly do. Clover honey is one of the most common types of honey available, and bees visit red clover throughout the summer and fall. The edible flowers are slightly sweet. You can pull the petals from the flower head and add them to salads throughout the summer. A few tiny florets are a delightful addition to a summer iced tea.

The raw greens of this plant are very nutritious, but like other members of the legume family (beans, peas), they are somewhat difficult to digest. The leaves are best enjoyed dried and in the tea form to get the nutrients and constituents without the side effects of gas and bloating common to eating legumes.

Red clover's constituents are thought to stimulate the immune system. (It has been a traditional ingredient in many formulas for cancer.) Red clover has also been used to treat coughs and respiratory system congestion, since it also contains resin. Resinous substances in plants have expectorating, warming, and antimicrobial action.

Red clover also contains the blood-thinning substance coumarin. Coumarin is not unique to red clover and is found in many other plants, including common grass. In fact, the pleasant sweet smell of freshly cut grass is due to the coumarin compounds.

SAW PALMETTO

Saw palmetto has long been considered an aphrodisiac and sexual rejuvenator, although little research supports the claim. Saw palmetto does act on the sexual organs, and many herbalists value it as a treatment for impotence. The action of saw palmetto has been well studied, and the herb is popular in the treatment of prostate enlargement. Enlargement of the prostate gland affects millions of men older than 50 years of age, causing difficulty with urination and a sensation of swelling in the low pelvis or rectal area. Research has shown that saw palmetto inhibits one of the active forms of testosterone in the body (dihydrotestosterone) from stimulating cellular reproduction in the prostate gland. Saw palmetto inhibits the binding of testosterone to prostate cells as well as the synthesis of testosterone. This serves to reduce multiplication of prostatic cells and reduces prostatic enlargement.

Saw palmetto is recommended to treat weakening urinary organs and the resulting incontinence that may occur in elderly people or women after menopause. Saw palmetto strengthens the urinary organs and has been recommended for kidney stones. Saw palmetto has also been touted as a steroid substitute for athletes who wish to increase muscle mass, though little documentation supports this claim. Saw palmetto does affect testosterone, one of the hormones responsible for promoting muscle mass, as described above, but the precise hormonal activities on tissues other than the prostate are not yet understood. Research on other plant steroids has shown their actions to be complex and diverse. Many plant steroids, for example, enhance hormonal activity in one type of tissue and inhibit it in others. The jury is out on whether saw palmetto will pump you up, but many herbalists agree that it may benefit cases of tissue wasting, weakness, debility, weight loss, and chronic emaciating diseases. However, this may be because saw palmetto improves digestion and absorption rather than producing any hormonal effect.

SHEPHERD'S PURSE

Shepherd's purse is used to stop heavy bleeding and hemorrhaging, particularly from the uterus. When taken internally, shepherd's purse can reduce heavy menstrual periods, and it has been used to treat postpartum hemorrhage. Still, it is considered most effective for the treatment of chronic uterine bleeding disorders, including uterine bleeding due to the presence of a fibroid tumor. Shepherd's purse has also been used internally to treat cases of blood in the urine and bleeding from the gastrointestinal tract such as with bleeding ulcers.

An astringent agent, shepherd's purse constricts blood vessels, thereby reducing blood flow. Shepherd's purse is also thought to cause the uterine muscle to contract, which also helps reduce bleeding. There have been reports that the hemostatic action (ability to stop bleeding) of shepherd's purse is not due to the plant itself, but due to a fungus that sometimes grows on the plant. This has not been proved. There is still much to learn about this herb.

When used topically, shepherd's purse is applied to lacerations and traumatic injuries of the skin to stop bleeding and promote healing. Herbalists also use the herb topically for eczema and rashes of the skin.

SKULLCAP

Skullcap is sometimes called mad dog in reference to its historical use in treating the symptoms of rabies, which can result from the bite of a rabid dog. Skullcap quiets nervous tension and eases muscle tension and spasms. Skullcap also induces sleep without strongly sedating or stupefying. Skullcap may help to lower elevated blood pressure.

Skullcap has been used for abnormally tense or twitching muscles, as occurs with rabies, Parkinson disease, St. Vitus dance (acute chorea, a nervous system disease characterized by involuntary movements of the limbs), and epilepsy.

Skullcap has also been found to have an anti-inflammatory action. Guinea pig studies have shown that skullcap also inhibits release of acetylcholine and histamine, two substances released by cells that cause inflammation.

SLIPPERY ELM

Added to water, the powdered bark becomes a soothing mucilage. The mucilage moistens and soothes while the herb's tannins are astringent, making slippery elm ideal to reduce inflammation and swelling, and heal damaged tissues. Mucilage is the most abundant constituent of slippery elm bark, but the tree also contains starch, sugar, calcium, iodine, bromine, amino acids, and traces of manganese and zinc. Many people eat slippery elm to soothe and nourish the body. Slippery elm helps heal internal mucosal tissues, such as the stomach, vagina, and esophagus. It is often recommended as a restorative herb for people who suffer from prolonged flu, stomach upset, chronic indigestion, and resulting malnutrition. You can use slippery elm to soothe ulcers and stomach inflammation, irritated intestines, vaginal inflammation, sore throat, coughs, and a hoarse voice.

ST. JOHN'S WORT

St. John's wort has long been used medicinally as an anti-inflammatory for strains, sprains, and contusions. St. John's wort also has been used to treat muscular spasms, cramps, and tension that results in muscular spasms.

The plant, especially its tiny yellow flowers, is high in hypericin and other flavonoid compounds. If you crush a flower bud between your fingers, you will release a burgundy red juice—evidence of the flavonoid hypericin. St. John's wort oils and tinctures should display this beautiful red coloring, which indicates the presence of the desired flavonoids. Bioflavonoids, in general, serve to reduce vascular fragility and inflammation. Since flavonoids improve venous-wall integrity, St. John's wort is useful in treating swollen veins.

St. John's wort preparations may be ingested for internal bruising and inflammation or following a traumatic injury to the external muscles and skin. The oil is also useful when applied to wounds and bruises or rubbed onto strains, sprains, or varicose veins. When rubbed onto the belly and breasts during pregnancy, the oil may also help prevent stretch marks. Topical application is also useful to treat hemorrhoids and aching, swollen veins that can occur during pregnancy.

St. John's wort is reported to relieve anxiety and tension and to act as an antidepressant. It was once thought that hypericin interferes with the body's production of a depression-related chemical called monoamine oxidase (MAO), but recent research has shed doubt on this claim. Though no one is yet certain how the herb works, studies have shown St. John's wort to act as a mood elevator in AIDS patients and in depressed subjects in general. The required dosage is three grams of powder per day, but it must be taken weeks and sometimes several months before results are noted.

St. John's wort is useful for pelvic pain and cramping. According to the 1983 British Pharmacopoeia, St. John's wort is specifically indicated for "menopausal neuroses": Many women who experience anxiety, depression, and other emotional disturbances during menopause may benefit from this herb's use. The National Cancer Institute has conducted several studies showing that St. John's wort has potential as a cancer-fighting drug. One study showed that mice injected with the feline leukemia virus were able to fight off the infection after just a single dose of St. John's wort.

UVA URSI

Uva ursi is used primarily to treat urinary problems, including bladder infections. The herb is disinfecting and promotes urine flow. Uva ursi is particularly recommended to treat illnesses caused by Escherichia coli (E. coli), a bacterium that lives in the intestines and commonly causes bladder and kidney infections. For kidney infections or kidney stones, take the herb under the care of a naturopathic or other trained physician. There is some indication that the herb may also be effective against certain yeast (such as Candida species).

Uva ursi is recommended for pelvic pain that is cramping, heavy, and dragging. The herb is particularly indicated for chronic complaints, although it should not be used over a long time. Use it for chronic irritation, pain, mucus production, and weakness of urinary organs

VALERIAN

Valerian is a lovely flowering plant used to relieve anxiety and relax muscles. Despite what some people have come to believe, valerian is not the source of the drug Valium, though it is an excellent sedative and hypnotic (sleep inducer). Valerian also has an antispasmodic action and is used for cramps, muscle pain, and muscle tension.
Valerian is commonly used for insomnia, tension, and nervousness. It's useful in simple cases of stress, anxiety, and nervous tension, as well as more severe cases of hysteria, nervous twitching, hyperactivity, chorea (involuntary jerky movements), heart palpitations, and tension headaches.

Valerian preparations are highly regarded for insomnia. Several studies show that valerian shortens the time needed to fall asleep and improves the quality of sleep. Unlike commonly used sedatives, valerian does not cause a drugged or hung-over sensation in most people.

The relaxing action of valerian also makes it useful for treatment of muscle cramps, menstrual cramps, and high blood pressure. Valerian relaxes the muscle in vein and artery walls and is especially indicated for elevated blood pressure due to stress and worry.

Valerian is used as a general nervine, meaning a substance that has a tonic effect on the nerves, restoring balance and relieving tension and anxiety. In the study of herbs, a nervine is classified as stimulating or sedating. Stimulating nervines are used in cases of sluggish mental activity, depression, or poor ability to concentrate, and sedating nervines are used to treat anxiety, turmoil, restlessness, and insomnia. Some herbalists consider valerian to be both stimulating and sedating, depending on the individual and the situation in which it is used. Occasionally, for example, people who use valerian to relax or improve sleep find that it worsens their complaints. Valerian is somewhat warming and stimulating, and perhaps the adverse reaction occurs in those who are already overly warm or stimulated. Valerian is best for treating depression caused by prolonged stress and nervous tension.

Valerian is mildly stimulating to the intestines, can help to dispel gas and cramps in the digestive tract, and is antimicrobial, particularly to bacteria.

WILD YAM

Dioscorea is a large genus that comprises more than 600 species. Wild yam's antispasmodic and anti-inflammatory properties make it useful to treat cramps in the stomach, intestines, and bile ducts, particularly the wavelike cramping pain caused by an intestinal virus or bacteria—what we might call stomach flu and colic in babies. Wild yam is also appropriate for flatulence and dysentery with cramps, especially if the conditions are caused by excess stomach acid.

The hormonal activity of wild yam has given it a reputation as a treatment for mentrual discomforts and premenstrual syndrome (PMS). A compound in yam, called diosgenin, is used as the basis for synthesizing several steroids, including progesterone and estrogen. However, this complicated process can be performed only in a laboratory, not in the body.

WORMWOOD

The most common use for this bitter herb is to stimulate the digestive system. You may be familiar with the practice of taking bitters before meals to aid digestion. A bitter taste in the mouth triggers release of bile from the gallbladder and other secretions from intestinal glands, which enables us to digest food.

People with weak digestion or insufficient stomach acid may benefit from taking wormwood preparations before meals. Wormwood, however, may cause diarrhea. Its secretion-stimulating qualities make the intestines empty quickly.

Because wormwood also contains a substance that is toxic if consumed for a long time, it is used only in small amounts for a short time.

Wormwood's bitter substances, called absinthin, have also been used to brew beer and distill alcohol. Absinthe, an old French liqueur prepared from wormwood, is now illegal because absinthol, a volatile oil the herb contains, has been found to cause nerve depression, mental impairment, and loss of reproductive function when used for a long time. Wormwood also lent its flavor and its name to vermouth. The German word for wormwood is Wermuth, which is the source of the modern word vermouth.

YARROW

Yarrow has been credited by scientists with at least minor activity on nearly every organ in the body. Early Greeks used the herb to stop hemorrhages. Yarrow was mentioned in Gerard's herbal in 1597 and many herbals thereafter. Yarrow was commonly used by Native American tribes for bleeding, wounds, and infections. It is used in Ayurvedic traditions, and traditional Chinese medicine credits yarrow with the ability to affect the spleen, liver, kidney, and bladder meridians, or energy channels, in the body.

Animal studies have supported the longstanding use of yarrow to cleanse wounds and control bleeding of lacerations, puncture wounds, and abrasions. Yarrow may also be used in tea or tincture form for bleeding ulcers, heavy menstrual periods, uterine hemorrhage, blood in the urine, or bleeding from the bowels. Yarrow compresses are effective for treating bleeding hemorrhoids.

Yarrow is often classified as a uterine tonic. Several studies have shown that yarrow can improve uterine tone, which may increase menstrual blood flow when it is irregular or scanty, and reduce uterine spasms, which reduces heavy flow in cases of abnormally heavy menstrual flow. In addition to its antispasmodic activity, the herb contains salicylic acid (a compound like the active ingredient in aspirin) and a volatile oil with anti-inflammatory properties, making it useful to relieve pain associated with gynecologic conditions, digestive disorders, and other conditions. Taken daily, yarrow preparations can relieve symptoms of menstrual cycle and uterine disorders such as cramps and endometriosis.

Yarrow also has antiseptic action against bacteria. The bitter constituents and fatty acids in yarrow are credited with promoting bile flow from the gallbladder, an action known as a cholagogue effect. Free-flowing bile enhances digestion and elimination and helps prevent gallstone formation. Because of these anti-inflammatory, antispasmodic, and cholagogue actions, yarrow is useful for gallbladder complaints and is considered a digestive tonic.

Yarrow has a drying effect and can be used as a decongestant. Sinus infections and coughs with sputum production may be improved by yarrow. Note, however, that a cough with ample sputum production may be a sign of bronchitis or pneumonia and require the attention of a physician. Yarrow's astringent action is also helpful in some cases of allergy, in which watery eyes and nasal secretions are triggered by pollen, dust, molds, and animal dander.

Yarrow also has long been used to promote sweating in cases of colds, flu, and fevers, thus helping you get over simple infections.

YELLOW DOCK

Yellow dock is commonly used as a laxative in cases of maldigestion (diminished ability to digest foods) and low stomach acid. Stomach acid helps dissolve the food you eat and break it down into simple chemical compounds the body can use. When there is a dysfunction in the digestive system, such as reduced stomach acid, your body is less able to absorb the protein and minerals in foods and to eliminate waste products. Yellow dock stimulates intestinal secretions, creating a mild laxative effect and helping to eliminate waste. It can also help bring stomach acids to normal levels. Yellow dock promotes the flow of bile from the liver and gallbladder, which appears to facilitate the absorption of minerals.

Like dandelion and burdock roots, yellow dock roots and preparations are used to improve conditions related to a sluggish digestive system, such as liver dysfunction, acne, headaches, and constipation. Because it improves absorption of nutrients, yellow dock is also used to treat anemia and poor hair, fingernail, and skin quality. All the docks are recommended for anemia resulting from an iron deficiency because, in addition to their ability to improve the absorption of iron from the intestines, they contain some iron. The docks are also high in bioflavonoids, which help strengthen capillaries.